Statistics for the Ophthalmologists
A Practical Guide

Statistics for the Ophthalmologists
A Practical Guide
Sankar Foundation Eye Hospital Manual for Understanding of Statistical Methods

Editors

T Raveendra MBBS MS FIGO FAICO
Director, CQI and Research
Head
Department of Anterior Segment and Glaucoma
Sankar Foundation Eye Hospital
Visakhapatnam, Andhra Pradesh, India

Sunil Moreker MBBS MS DOMS
Associate Professor
Department of Ophthalmology
MGM Medical College
Navi Mumbai, Maharashtra, India

Krishna Prasad Pallem MBBS MS DO
Professor
Department of Medical Education
Sankar Foundation Eye Hospital
Visakhapatnam, Andhra Pradesh, India

Forewords

Namrata Sharma
B Muniswamy

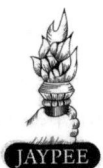

JAYPEE BROTHERS MEDICAL PUBLISHERS
The Health Sciences Publisher
New Delhi | London

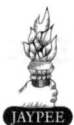 **Jaypee Brothers Medical Publishers (P) Ltd**

Headquarters
EMCA House, 23/23-B
Ansari Road, Daryaganj
New Delhi 110 002, India
Landline: +91-11-23272143, +91-11-23272703
+91-11-23282021, +91-11-23245672
e-mail: jaypee@jaypeebrothers.com

Corporate Office
4838/24, Ansari Road, Daryaganj
New Delhi 110 002, India
Phone: +91-11-43574357
Fax: +91-11-43574314
e-mail: jaypee@jaypeebrothers.com

Overseas Office
JP Medical Ltd.
83, Victoria Street, London
SW1H 0HW (UK)
Phone: +44-20 3170 8910
e-mail: info@jpmedpub.com

EU GPSR Authorised Representative
Logos Europe, 9 rue Nicolas Poussin
17000, La Rochelle, France
Phone: +33 (0) 6 67 93 73 78
e-mail: contact@logoseurope.eu

Website: www.jaypeebrothers.com
Website: www.jaypeedigital.com

© 2026, Jaypee Brothers Medical Publishers

The views and opinions expressed in this book are solely those of the original contributor(s)/author(s) and do not necessarily represent those of editor(s) or publisher of the book.

All rights reserved. No part of this publication may be reproduced, stored or transmitted in any form or by any means, electronic, mechanical, photocopying, recording or otherwise, without the prior permission in writing of the publishers.

All brand names and product names used in this book are trade names, service marks, trademarks or registered trademarks of their respective owners. The publisher is not associated with any product or vendor mentioned in this book.

Medical knowledge and practice change constantly. This book is designed to provide accurate, authoritative information about the subject matter in question. However, readers are advised to check the most current information available on procedures included and check information from the manufacturer of each product to be administered, to verify the recommended dose, formula, method and duration of administration, adverse effects and contra indications. It is the responsibility of the practitioner to take all appropriate safety precautions. Neither the publisher nor the author(s)/editor(s) assume any liability for any injury and/or damage to persons or property arising from or related to use of material in this book.

This book is sold on the understanding that the publisher is not engaged in providing professional medical services. If such advice or services are required, the services of a competent medical professional should be sought.

Every effort has been made where necessary to contact holders of copyright to obtain permission to reproduce copyright material. If any have been inadvertently overlooked, the publisher will be pleased to make the necessary arrangements at the first opportunity.

Inquiries for bulk sales may be solicited at: jaypee@jaypeebrothers.com

Statistics for the Ophthalmologists: A Practical Guide

First Edition: **2026**

ISBN: 978-93-6616-139-6

Printed in India

Dedicated to

Shri Atmakuri Sankar Rao (September 2, 1931–March 18, 2012).

The Founder Trustee, whose vision and dedication have been the cornerstone of our journey. His unwavering support and guidance have been instrumental in shaping our path and inspiring us to strive for excellence.

This book is a testament to his enduring legacy and commitment to advancing the field of ophthalmology.

Contributors

Ajay Sharma
MBBS MS FVRS
Director
Vitreoretinal Services
Sankar Foundation Eye Hospital
Visakhapatnam, Andhra Pradesh, India

Annaji Rao Kota
MBBS DNB
Senior Consultant
Department of Retina
Sankar Foundation Eye Hospital
Visakhapatnam, Andhra Pradesh, India

B Muniswami
PhD (Statistics)
Head
Department of Statistics
Honorary Director
Population Research Centre
Andhra University
Visakhapatnam, Andhra Pradesh, India

B Punyavathi
PhD (Statistics)
Guest Faculty
Department of Statistics
Andhra University
Visakhapatnam, Andhra Pradesh, India

Bhanu Boddi
MBBS DNB
Junior Consultant
Department of Cornea
Sankar Foundation Eye Hospital
Visakhapatnam, Andhra Pradesh, India

Ditsha Datta
MBBS MS
Fellow
Department of Glaucoma
Sankar Foundation Eye Hospital
Visakhapatnam, Andhra Pradesh, India

Durga Bhavani Mummina
MSc (Statistics)
Research Associate
Department of Research and Development
Sankar Foundation Eye Hospital
Visakhapatnam, Andhra Pradesh, India

Jagannadha Kumar Challa
MBBS FIVRS
Senior Retina Consultant
Department of Retina
Sankar Foundation Eye Hospital
Visakhapatnam, Andhra Pradesh, India

Jaya Siresha Nakka
MBBS DO Fellowship in Orbit Oculoplasty
Head
Department of Orbit Oculoplasty
Sankar Foundation Eye Hospital
Visakhapatnam, Andhra Pradesh, India

Kavithadevi Mamchimsetti
MBBS MS
Senior Consultant
Department of Glaucoma
Sankar Foundation Eye Hospital
Visakhapatnam, Andhra Pradesh, India

Keerthana Bonsi
MBBS MS
Junior Consultant
Department of Glaucoma
Sankar Foundation Eye Hospital
Visakhapatnam, Andhra Pradesh, India

Krishna Prasad Pallem
MBBS MS DO
Professor
Department of Medical Education
Sankar Foundation Eye Hospital
Visakhapatnam, Andhra Pradesh, India

Krishna Talabhaktula
MBBS DO
Head
Department of Retina
Sankar Foundation Eye Hospital
Visakhapatnam, Andhra Pradesh, India

Manju Valli Pavuluri
MBBS MS
Senior Consultant
Department of Glaucoma
Sankar Foundation Eye Hospital
Visakhapatnam, Andhra Pradesh, India

Nasrin
MBBS DO DNB FICS
Director
Medical Administration and Training
Sankar Foundation Eye Hospital
Visakhapatnam, Andhra Pradesh, India

Sowmya Peri
MBBS DNB
Senior Consultant
Department of Cornea
Sankar Foundation Eye Hospital
Visakhapatnam, Andhra Pradesh, India

Srinivasa Rao Pasala
PhD (Statistics)
Assistant Professor
Department of Statistics
Gayatri Vidya Parishad (A) College for Degree and PG Courses
Visakhapatnam, Andhra Pradesh, India

Sunil Moreker
MBBS MS DOMS
Associate Professor
Department of Ophthalmology
MGM Medical College
Navi Mumbai, Maharashtra, India

Suparna G
MBBS DO FIPOS
Head
Department of Pediatric Ophthalmology
Sankar Foundation Eye Hospital
Visakhapatnam, Andhra Pradesh, India

T Raveendra
MBBS MS FIGO FAICO
Director, CQI and Research
Head
Department of Anterior Segment and Glaucoma
Sankar Foundation Eye Hospital
Visakhapatnam, Andhra Pradesh, India

Veerendra Babu Odugu
MSc (Statistics) PhD
Assistant Professor
Department of Statistics
School of Advanced Sciences
Vellore Institute of Technology
Vellore, Tamil Nadu, India

Foreword

As an ophthalmologist, it is a pleasure to introduce *Statistics for the Ophthalmologists: A Practical Guide*, which bridges clinical expertise and statistical science. I admire the precision and dedication required in our field, and this book, enhanced by a biostatistician, addresses the complexity of statistical methods head-on, making them accessible and relevant to ophthalmology.

The book's practical approach, with real-world examples and case studies, highlights the significant role of statistics in clinical practice. Sections on published literature delve into advanced topics, providing deeper insights that are crucial for our understanding.

Statistics for the Ophthalmologists: A Practical Guide is a great resource for ophthalmologists across all levels of expertise. It empowers us to navigate statistical data confidently and fosters informed and effective practice. I commend the authors for their exceptional work and believe that this book will be a cornerstone of ophthalmologic education and practice.

Namrata Sharma MD
Professor
Department of Ophthalmology
Dr Rajendra Prasad Centre for Ophthalmic Sciences
All India Institute of Medical Sciences
New Delhi, India

Foreword

It is a pleasure to introduce *Statistics for the Ophthalmologists: A Practical Guide*, which bridges clinical expertise and statistical science. As a senior statistician, I admire the precision and dedication of ophthalmologists. This book, enhanced by a biostatistician, addresses the complexity of statistical methods head-on, making them accessible and relevant to the field.

The book's practical approach, with real-world examples and case studies, highlights the role of statistics in clinical practice. Sections on published literature delve into advanced topics, providing deeper insights.

Statistics for the Ophthalmologists: A Practical Guide hopefully will prove to be a great resource for ophthalmologists across the levels of expertise, empowering them to navigate statistical data and fostering informed and effective practice. I commend the authors for their exceptional work and believe that this book will be a cornerstone of ophthalmologic education and practice.

B Muniswamy PhD (Statistics)
Head
Department of Statistics
Honorary Director
Population Research Centre
Andhra University
Visakhapatnam, Andhra Pradesh, India

Preface

In the realm of ophthalmology, understanding statistical concepts is paramount for both clinical and research purposes. This book *Statistics for the Ophthalmologists: A Practical Guide* was born out of the necessity to bridge the gap between complex statistical jargon and its practical application in the field of eye care.

We recognize that the language of statistics can often seem impenetrable, with its myriad of terms, formulas, and theoretical underpinnings. For many practitioners, these concepts remain elusive, which can hinder the interpretation of research findings and the application of evidence-based practices.

Our goal with this guide is to demystify statistics and present it in a way that is accessible and relevant to ophthalmologists. Through clear explanations, practical examples, and a focus on real-world applications, we aim to make statistical principles not only understandable but also useful in everyday practice.

We hope that this book will serve as a valuable resource, helping ophthalmologists to confidently navigate the statistical aspects of their work and ultimately improve patient outcomes.

T Raveendra
Sunil Moreker
Krishna Prasad Pallem

Acknowledgments

We extend our heartfelt gratitude to the trustees of Sankar Foundation, Visakhapatnam, Andhra Pradesh, India represented by A Krishna Kumar, for their unwavering support and vision that have been the driving force behind this project. We are immensely grateful to Sri K Radhakrishnan, GM, Sankar Foundation, for his continued encouragement and resources that have made this guide possible.

Special thanks go to the dedicated doctors, fellows, and DNB residents whose invaluable contributions and tireless efforts have enriched this book. Their commitment to excellence in ophthalmology and relentless pursuit of knowledge have been truly inspiring.

We also wish to acknowledge all the staff of Sankar Foundation for their hard work and dedication, which have been crucial in the development and completion of this guide. Your collective efforts have significantly enhanced its quality and impact.

A special acknowledgment extends to Professor (Dr) Namrata Sharma, Department of Ophthalmology, Dr Rajendra Prasad Centre for Ophthalmic Sciences, All India Institute of Medical Sciences, New Delhi, and Professor (Dr) B Muniswami, Head, Department of Statistics, Andhra University, Visakhapatnam, Andhra Pradesh, whose expertise, insights, and unwavering support and forewords have been instrumental in shaping this book. Their contributions have been indispensable, and we are deeply appreciative of their involvement.

Finally, we would like to thank Shri Jitendar P Vij (Group Chairman), Mr Ankit Vij (Managing Director), Mr MS Mani (Group President), Bikram Sardar (Commissioning Editor), Pratiksha Dubey (Development Editor) of M/s Jaypee Brothers Medical Publishers (P) Ltd, New Delhi, India and many others, for their professional and dedicated support throughout this process. Their assistance has been invaluable, and we are grateful for their partnership.

This book would not have been possible without the collective efforts and dedication of all these individuals and organizations. We are profoundly grateful for your contributions and support.

Contents

1. **Introduction** 1
   Jagannadha Kumar Challa, Krishna Prasad Pallem, Srinivasa Rao Pasala

2. **Basic Concepts and Statistical Tools** 12
   T Raveendra, Ditsha Datta, B Muniswami

3. **Data Collection Techniques** 21
   Nasrin, Bhanu Boddi, Durga Bhavani Mummina

4. **Sampling Techniques** 30
   Krishna Prasad Pallem, B Muniswami

5. **Charts and Graphs** 42
   Sunil Moreker, Keerthana Bonsi, B Punyavathi

6. **Measures of Central Tendency** 53
   Nasrin, Jaya Siresha Nakka, Durga Bhavani Mummina

7. **Measures of Dispersion** 69
   Suparna G, B Punyavathi

8. **Probability and Distributions** 81
   Sunil Moreker, T Raveendra, Srinivasa Rao Pasala, Sowmya Peri

9. **Correlation and Regression** 90
   Krishna Prasad Pallem, Srinivasa Rao Pasala

10. **Inferential Statistics** 104
    T Raveendra, Annaji Rao Kota, Durga Bhavani Mummina

11. **Sample Size Determination** 143
    Ajay Sharma, Durga Bhavani Mummina

12. **Tools in Data Analysis** 161
    Ajay Sharma, T Raveendra, Veerendra Babu Odugu

13. **Role of Artificial Intelligence in Ophthalmic Statistics** 173
    T Raveendra, Manju Valli Pavuluri, B Punyavathi

14. **Collaboration with Biostatistician** 183
    Krishna Talabhaktula, Kavithadevi Mamchimsetti, B Punyavathi

Appendices

1. **Research Frameworks in Clinical Ophthalmology** 193
   T Raveendra, B Muniswami

2. **Research Project Flow: From Idea to Innovation** 212
   Sunil Moreker, Ditsha Datta

Index *217*

CHAPTER 1

Introduction

Jagannadha Kumar Challa, Krishna Prasad Pallem, Srinivasa Rao Pasala

■ INTRODUCTION

Ophthalmology is not only a beautiful field that delicately intertwines the art of vision care with the precision of medical science but also a domain where the harmonious blend of statistics and artificial intelligence can propel the boundaries of what is possible. The intricate dance between these disciplines highlights the necessity for interdisciplinary collaboration, envisioning a future where the clinician-scientist and every clinician of tomorrow are well versed in both the clinical and analytical realms.

In ophthalmology, the use of statistical methods, AI technologies, and ethical considerations is crucial for clinical practice and research advancement. Despite significant progress, there remain notable gaps in knowledge that necessitate a keen focus on study design and the interpretation of clinical research.

■ CLINICIAN, CLINICIAN–SCIENTIST, AND HOLISTIC CLINICIAN

The Clinician, Clinician–Scientist, and Holistic Clinician are essential roles in the evolving landscape of healthcare. Each brings a unique perspective and skill set that, when integrated, can propel medical advancements to new heights **(Fig. 1.1)**.

Clinician

A *clinician* is a healthcare professional who is directly involved in patient care. This includes doctors, nurses, therapists, and other medical practitioners who diagnose, treat, and manage patients' health conditions. Clinicians work in various settings such as hospitals, clinics, and private practices.

Clinician–Scientist

A *clinician-scientist* (or physician-scientist) is a medical professional who combines clinical practice with scientific research. They spend part of their time treating patients and the other part conducting research to advance medical knowledge and improve patient care **(Table 1.1)**. Clinician–scientists often hold both medical and research degrees (e.g., MD-PhD) and work in academic or research institutions.

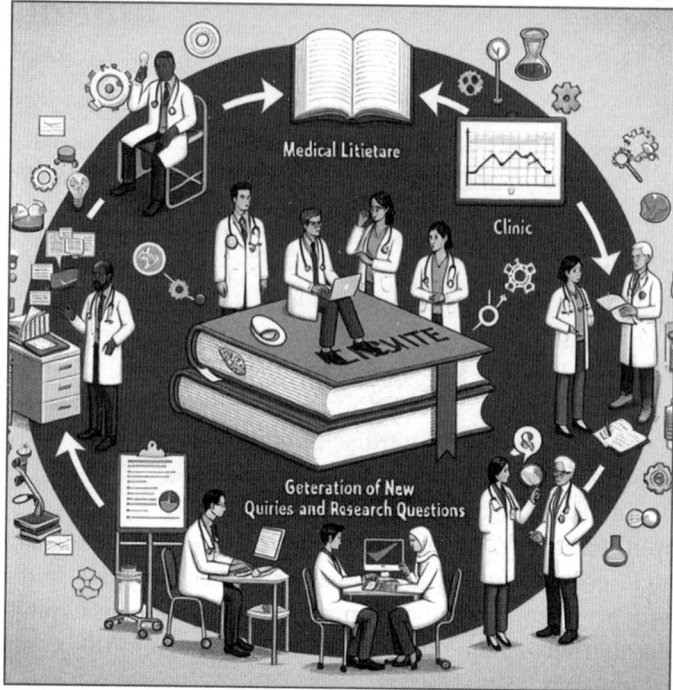

Fig. 1.1: The cycle of refinement of knowledge and practice patterns in clinical sciences.
(*Source:* This image is an AI-generated illustration created using DALL-E 3)

TABLE 1.1: The holistic clinician's checklist	
Issue	*Details*
Jumping to *p*-value	Leads to misinterpretations in research
Magnitude or clinical relevance	*p*-value alone does not provide this information
Confidence intervals	Offer insights into precision and reliability
Study design and data interpretation	Consideration of confounding variables and robustness of analytical methods
Erroneous conclusions	Can lead to misleading information in the medical community
Holistic approach	Combines statistical principles with clinical expertise
Proper interpretation	Includes *p*-values, confidence intervals, and effect sizes
Informed decisions	Improves patient care and advances ophthalmology

Holistic Clinician

A *holistic clinician* focuses on treating the whole person—body, mind, spirit, and emotions—rather than just addressing specific symptoms or diseases. They use a combination of conventional medical treatments and alternative therapies to promote overall wellbeing. Holistic clinicians may include doctors of osteopathy, naturopaths, chiropractors, and other practitioners who emphasize a balanced approach to health.

A holistic clinician is one who transcends traditional boundaries, integrating a deep understanding of clinical aspects with advanced analytical skills in biostatistics and artificial intelligence; there will be an understanding requirement on ethical aspects too.

Such a clinician recognizes that the future of healthcare depends on the ability to leverage interdisciplinary knowledge to address complex medical challenges. In the context of ophthalmology, this means being sufficiently proficient in the applicable ethical aspects, statistical methodologies, and possibly the AI techniques to enhance both patient care and research outcomes.

The holistic clinician embodies a commitment to continuous learning, staying updated with emerging trends and innovations that can be applied to clinical practice. This approach not only improves diagnostic and therapeutic strategies but also fosters a collaborative environment where diverse expertise converges to push the frontiers of medical science.

Illustration

Imagine an ophthalmologist studying the effectiveness of a new eye drop treatment for dry eye syndrome. To ensure the study is statistically robust, they collaborate with a biostatistician. The biostatistician helps design the study, determining the sample size needed to detect a significant effect and advising on randomization methods to reduce bias. They also assist in analyzing the collected data, using statistical tests to compare the treatment group with a control group. This collaboration ensures that the study's findings are valid and reliable, providing clear evidence on the treatment's efficacy.

Consider a clinical situation where an ophthalmologist encounters a patient with a rare retinal disease showing progressive visual deterioration. The holistic clinician, equipped with knowledge in AI and biostatistics, formulates a research question: "What are the predictive factors for the progression of this rare retinal disease based on imaging and genetic data?"

To address this question, the clinician collaborates with biostatisticians and data scientists to design a methodologically sound study. They utilize machine learning algorithms to analyze a comprehensive dataset comprising retinal images, genetic sequences, and patient health records. Through this interdisciplinary approach, they identify key biomarkers and patterns that predict disease progression, ultimately leading to more personalized and effective treatment strategies.

TRANSITION FROM KNOWLEDGE GAP TO KNOWLEDGE APPLICATION

One critical gap in knowledge pertains to the variability in study designs used in ophthalmic research. A comprehensive understanding of various study designs, including randomized controlled trials, cohort studies, and case-control studies, is imperative for ophthalmologists to draw valid conclusions from their investigations. Each study design has its strengths and limitations, and their appropriate application can significantly impact the reliability of research findings.

Moreover, the interpretation of statistical results in ophthalmology demands a thorough grasp of biostatistical principles. Ophthalmologists must be adept at interpreting p-values, confidence intervals, and regression analyses within the context of their specific research questions. Misinterpretation of statistical data can lead to erroneous conclusions and potentially compromise patient care.

RESEARCH METHODOLOGY, STATISTICAL ANALYSIS, AND ETHICS—IMPORTANCE OF SEPARATE FOCUS SESSIONS

Research methodology (RM), statistical analysis (SA), and ethical standards are three critical components of scientific research, each with distinct roles and responsibilities. Understanding the nuances of RM and SA is crucial for conducting robust and reliable research. This document delineates the key differences between RM and SA; and illustrates the importance of having separate focus sessions for each, rather than combining them into a single session.

Research Methodology

Research methodology encompasses the strategies, techniques, and tools used to design and conduct research. It involves planning and structuring the entire research process, from formulating a hypothesis to collecting data. Key aspects of RM include:
- *Study design:* Determining the appropriate type of study (e.g., experimental, observational, and longitudinal) based on the research question.

- *Sampling methods:* Selecting a representative sample from the population to ensure generalizability of the results.
- *Data collection:* Choosing the right data collection methods (e.g., surveys, experiments, and interviews) and tools (e.g., questionnaires and sensors).
- *Ethical considerations:* Ensuring the study adheres to ethical guidelines and obtains necessary approvals.
- *Operational definitions:* Clearly defining variables and ensuring they are measured consistently.

Research methodology is the blueprint of research, guiding researchers through the process, and ensuring that the study is methodologically sound and capable of addressing the research questions effectively.

Statistical Analysis

Statistical analysis, on the other hand, focuses on the examination and interpretation of the collected data. It involves applying statistical techniques to analyze data and draw meaningful conclusions. Key aspects of SA include:
- *Descriptive statistics:* Summarizing data using measures such as mean, median, mode, standard deviation, and frequency distributions
- *Inferential statistics:* Making predictions or inferences about a population based on sample data, using techniques such as hypothesis testing, confidence intervals, and regression analysis
- *Data visualization:* Creating graphs, charts, and plots to visually represent the data and identify patterns or trends.
- *Modeling and simulation:* Developing statistical models to describe relationships between variables and simulate potential outcomes.
- *Assumptions checking:* Ensuring that the data meet the assumptions required for the chosen statistical tests.

Statistical analysis is the process of making sense of the data, providing empirical evidence to support or refute hypotheses and enabling researchers to draw valid conclusions.

The Need for Separate Focus Sessions

While RM and SA are interrelated and both essential for conducting research, they require distinct skill sets and knowledge bases. Here are some reasons why it is beneficial to have separate focus sessions for RM and SA:
- *Depth of coverage:* Each area is vast and complex, warranting in-depth exploration. Separate sessions allow for a comprehensive examination of each topic, ensuring that essential concepts and techniques are thoroughly covered.
- *Focus on specific skills:* RM involves skills related to study design, sampling, and data collection, while SA requires expertise in statistical techniques

and data interpretation. Separate sessions allow participants to develop and hone these specific skills independently.
- *Tailored learning:* Researchers may have varying levels of proficiency in RM and SA. Separate sessions enable instructors to tailor the content to the participants' needs, providing targeted training and addressing specific knowledge gaps.
- *Reduced cognitive load:* Combining RM and SA into a single session can be overwhelming, as it requires assimilating a large amount of information from different domains. Separate sessions reduce cognitive load, making it easier for participants to absorb and retain the material.

Ethical Aspects Overview

Ethical considerations play a pivotal role in RM and SA. Proper adherence to ethical guidelines ensures the integrity and validity of research findings.

Key ethical aspects include obtaining informed consent from participants, ensuring confidentiality and privacy, avoiding conflicts of interest, and maintaining transparency in data reporting. Researchers must also be vigilant about the ethical implications of their study design and data interpretation, avoiding practices such as p-hacking and selective reporting.

By adhering to these ethical standards, clinicians enhance the credibility and reliability of their work and research. This, in turn, fosters trust while delivering services and advancing knowledge within their respective fields.

■ INTERDISCIPLINARY COLLABORATION ENHANCES VALUE

Interdisciplinary collaboration between clinicians and other fields is important for potential advancements. Ophthalmologists, biostatisticians, and data scientists must work together to design studies that are methodologically sound and analytically robust. This collaboration ensures that the research addresses clinically relevant questions and that the findings are translating to real-world settings.

Ophthalmology, as a specialized branch of medicine, frequently encounters complex data sets derived from imaging, genetic sequencing, and patient health records. The application of AI, particularly machine learning and deep learning, holds the promise of uncovering patterns and insights that were previously obscured. However, the successful implementation of these techniques is contingent upon well-designed studies that accurately capture the nuances of ophthalmic conditions.

Furthermore, the dynamic nature of ophthalmic research necessitates ongoing education and training in the basics and advances in statistical techniques and even the AI-related advances. Continuous professional development enables ophthalmologists to stay abreast of emerging trends and to apply cutting-edge methodologies in their practice.

Insights into Collaborating Disciplines

Understanding various depths of collaborating disciplines is crucial in the realm of ophthalmology, as it enables a holistic approach to addressing complex clinical and research challenges. Each discipline brings its unique perspectives, methodologies, and expertise, which are essential for comprehensive problem-solving. By delving into the intricacies of related fields such as biostatistics, data science, and artificial intelligence, ophthalmologists can enhance their clinical practice and research capabilities.

This interdisciplinary knowledge allows for the design of robust studies that yield reliable and clinically relevant results. For instance, a thorough understanding of biostatistical principles helps ophthalmologists interpret data accurately and avoid common pitfalls such as misinterpreting p-values or correlation coefficients. Similarly, insights into AI techniques enable the application of advanced analytical tools to uncover patterns and trends in complex datasets, leading to more informed clinical decisions.

Furthermore, interdisciplinary collaboration fosters innovation and the development of novel solutions that push the boundaries of what is possible in ophthalmic care. By working closely with experts from various fields, ophthalmologists can stay abreast of emerging trends and technologies, ensuring they are well-equipped to tackle the evolving challenges in their practice.

In conclusion, having insights of various depths into collaborating disciplines is imperative for advancing ophthalmology. It promotes rigorous study design, accurate data interpretation, and innovative problem-solving, ultimately enhancing clinical outcomes and contributing to the growing body of medical knowledge.

In conclusion, although advancements advanced statistical methods and artificial intelligence hold significant potential to transform ophthalmic research and practice patterns, it is essential to bridge the knowledge gaps in study design and data interpretation. Achieving this requires a sufficient level of interdisciplinary expertise and insightful knowledge.

The Benefits are Mutual and Wide Reaching

By embracing an interdisciplinary approach, clinicians can gain deeper insights into the methodologies and analytical frameworks used by biostatisticians and AI scientists, leading to more effective collaboration and innovation. This mutual understanding fosters a culture of continuous learning and improvement, where each discipline's expertise is harnessed to address complex ophthalmic challenges.

Similarly, biostatisticians and AI scientists stand to benefit from collaborating with clinicians, as it provides them with a practical understanding of the clinical context and the nuances of ophthalmic conditions. This knowledge is crucial for developing and refining analytical tools and models that are both clinically relevant and robust.

By fostering such interdisciplinary collaboration and prioritizing rigorous study designs, the field of ophthalmology can leverage these powerful tools to enhance clinical outcomes and contribute to the evolving body of medical knowledge for the benefits to various disciplines and ultimately to the whole society.

■ HOLISTIC CLINICIAN'S RULEBOOK AND CHECKLIST

The journey to be a holistic clinician is long but nevertheless necessary and feasible. One of the reasons being that the data in our face are to be interpreted effectively for the expectations of the patient and there may not be any clear shortcut; the rules of the journey are therefore to be defined. Let us look at an example to start with while contemplating to generalize with a set of rules.

The tendency of jumping straight to the p-value can lead to significant misinterpretations in research. It is crucial to avoid this practice for several reasons.

First, a *p-value* alone does not provide information about the magnitude or clinical relevance of an effect, which can result in overestimating the importance of statistically significant findings.

Second, relying solely on p-values neglects the context of *confidence intervals*, which offer essential insights into the precision and reliability of the estimated effect.

Additionally, a singular focus on p-values can overshadow other critical aspects of *study design and data interpretation*, such as the consideration of *confounding variables* and the *robustness of the analytical methods* used. This approach can lead to erroneous conclusions and the propagation of misleading information within the medical community.

By fostering a comprehensive understanding of statistical principles and integrating them with clinical expertise, we can enhance the quality of ophthalmic research. Properly interpreting statistical results, including p-values, confidence intervals, and effect sizes, ensures that the findings are both statistically and clinically meaningful. This holistic approach helps in making informed decisions, ultimately improving patient care and advancing the field of ophthalmology.

Examples of Avoidable Follies

There have been notable instances where misinterpretation of statistical parameters has led to erroneous conclusions in ophthalmic research. For example, a study that employed p-values without considering confidence intervals might suggest a statistically significant effect that is not clinically meaningful. Misinterpreting the *p*-value as an indication of the size of an effect, rather than merely its statistical significance, can mislead researchers about the true efficacy of a treatment.

It may look good as an initial impression that a study of the 2.2-mm microincision cataract surgery offers a lower and more stable SIA compared to the 3.0-mm incision. The clinical significance, however, may include other aspects to be undertaken and taken cognizance, such as Descemet's membrane detachment, effects on endothelial cell counts, and patient reported outcomes.

Another instance is the misuse of correlation coefficients. A high correlation between two variables does not imply causation, yet some studies have drawn causal inferences from mere associations. For example, a study may report a high correlation between ocular pressure and a specific medication without considering other confounding variables, leading to incorrect assumptions about the medication's direct effect on ocular pressure.

The article by (Lu et al., 2022/03/03) on the study of peripapillary choroidal vascularity and visual correlates in nonarteritic anterior ischemic optic neuropathy using swept-source optical coherence tomography, employs Bonferroni-corrected values after initial correlations. They use Bonferroni correction to adjust for multiple comparisons and reduce the risk of type I errors (false positive), ensuring that the findings are statistically significant **(Table 1.2)**.

The inappropriate use of multiple comparisons without proper correction methods, such as the Bonferroni correction, can lead to false positives. In ophthalmology, where multiple outcomes might be assessed from imaging data, failing to adjust for multiple testing increases the risk of finding *spurious associations* that do not hold up under rigorous scrutiny.

These examples underscore the importance of proper statistical training and interdisciplinary collaboration to prevent the propagation of flawed research findings. By ensuring that studies are methodologically sound and that statistical analyses are correctly interpreted, the field of ophthalmology can avoid these pitfalls and advance with robust and reliable research.

■ CONCLUSION

Research methodology and SA are both fundamental to the research process, but they encompass distinct aspects that require focused attention. By conducting separate sessions for RM and SA, researchers can gain a deeper understanding of each area, develop specific skills, and ultimately conduct more robust and reliable studies. This approach not only enhances the quality of research but also fosters effective collaboration among interdisciplinary teams.

TABLE 1.2: Study applying Bonferroni correction to reduce risks of type I (false positive error).

	NAION eyes (n = 17)	Fellow eyes (n = 6)	Control eyes (n = 18)	p-value, NAION vs. control	p-value, fellow vs. control	p-value, NAION vs. fellow
Age, years	62.8 ± 9.4	59.2 ± 9.0	60.5 ± 5.5	>0.99	>0.99	>0.99
Sex, male (%)	13 (76.5)	6 (100)	13 (72.2)	>0.99	0.50	0.73
BCVA, LogMAR	0.12 ± 03	−0.02 ± 0.1	0.02 ± 0.1	0.30	>0.99	0.35
IOP, mm Hg	15.0 ± 2.2	15.6 ± 2.9	15.8 ± 3.0	>0.99	>0.99	>0.99
HVF mean deviation, dB	−13.1 ± 7.3	−0.5 ± 1.5	N/A	N/A	N/A	<0.001*
HVF pattern standard deviation dB	11.7 ± 4.7	1.5 ± 0.3	N/A	N/A	N/A	<0.001*
Mean PCT, μm	278.0 ± 65.2	221.4 ± 50.4	157.5 ± 26.9	<0.001*	0.028*	0.063
Superior quadrant PCT, μm	278.8 ± 77.0	215.6 ± 61.7	150.2 ± 27.0	<0.001*	0.063	0.08
Inferior quadrant PCT, μm	263.3 ± 90.5	205.5 ± 58.9	135.8 ± 36.2	<0.001*	0.10	0.23
Nasal quadrant PCT, μm	278.1 ± 58.8	226.1 ± 51.1	175.9 ± 27.7	<0.001*	0.082	0.069
Temporal quadrant PCT, μm	291.7 ± 76.0	238.6 ± 50.8	167.9 ± 33.5	<0.001*	0.038*	0.173
Mean CVI	035 ± 0.03	0.35 ± 0.04	038 ± 0.02	<0.008*	0.068	>0.99
Nasal CVI	038 ± 0.03	0.38 ± 0.02	0.40 ± 0.02	0.035*	0.65	>0.99
Temporal CVI	033 ± 0.04	0.32 ± 0.06	037 ± 0.04	0.048*	0.095	>0.99

(BCVA: best-corrected visual acuity; CVI: choroidal vascularity index; HVF: Humphrey visual field; JOP: intraocular pressure; LogMAR: logarithm of the minimum angle of resolution; NAJON: nonarteritic anterior ischemic optic neuropathy; PCT: peripapillary choroidal thickness; SS-OCT: swept-source optical coherence tomography)

Values presented as mean ± standard deviation unless otherwise noted.

*Indicates $p < 0.05$. Bonferroni-corrected pairwise comparisons

■ BIBLIOGRAPHY

1. Liang JL, Xing XL, Yang XT, Jiang YF, Zhang H. Clinical comparison analysis in surgically induced astigmatism of the total, anterior and posterior cornea after 2.2-mm versus 3.0-mm clear corneal incision cataract surgery. Zhonghua Yan Ke Za Zhi [Internet]. 2019 (cited 07/11/2019);55(7):495-501. Available from: https://doi.org/10.3760/cma.j.issn.0412-4081.2019.07.004
2. Lu ES, Katz R, Miller JB, Gaier ED. Peripapillary choroidal vascularity and visual correlates in non-arteritic anterior ischemic optic neuropathy using swept-source optical coherence tomography. Front Ophthalmol (Lausanne) [Internet]. 2022 (cited 03/03/2022);2:848040. Available from: https://doi.org/10.3389/fopht.2022.848040

Basic Concepts and Statistical Tools

CHAPTER 2

T Raveendra, Ditsha Datta, B Muniswami

■ INTRODUCTION

In the realm of statistics, understanding the various types of data is fundamental to conducting effective analysis and drawing meaningful conclusions. Data, in its essence, is the raw information collected from observations, measurements, or experiments, and it can be classified into distinct categories based on its characteristics and the level of measurement it entails.

The primary classification of data in statistics encompasses four main types—(1) nominal, (2) ordinal, (3) interval, and (4) ratio **(Flowchart 2.1)**. Each type of data possesses unique properties and serves specific purposes in the interpretation and analysis of statistical information.

Nominal data represents the most basic level of data measurement, characterized by categories or labels that signify distinct groups without any particular order or ranking. It is commonly used in fields such as ophthalmology to categorize variables such as eye color, types of eye diseases, patient gender, and blood type. This type of data is purely qualitative and is useful for identifying, classifying, and summarizing information into discrete groups.

Understanding the intricacies of these data types is crucial for statistical analysis, as it allows researchers and analysts to select appropriate methods

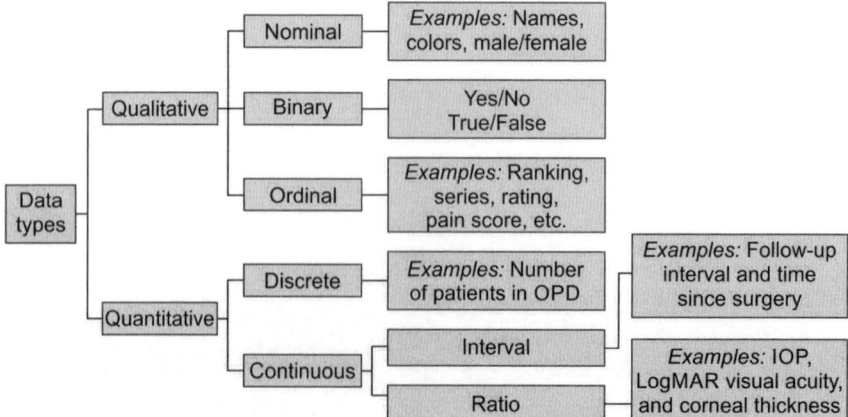

Flowchart 2.1: Data and its classification.

and techniques for data collection, processing, and interpretation. In the following sections, we will delve deeper into each type of data, exploring their characteristics and applications in various fields, with a particular emphasis on their relevance in ophthalmology.

Continuous data in the ratio type is considered the most powerful level in measurement of data in statistics **(Table 2.1)**. This is because ratio data not only incorporates all the properties of nominal, ordinal, and interval data, but it also has a true zero point, which allows for the calculation of meaningful ratios. This level of data enables a wide range of statistical analyses, including measures of central tendency and variability, correlation, and regression analyses. In medical research including ophthalmology, ratio data can be crucial for precise measurements, such as intraocular pressure, visual acuity, and other quantifiable factors that inform diagnosis and treatment.

■ DATA AND ITS TYPES

In statistics, data can be classified into two types—(1) qualitative and (2) quantitative data which can be classified into four subtypes—(1) nominal, (2) ordinal, (3) interval, and (4) ratio.

Qualitative Data

Qualitative data, also known as categorical data, is descriptive and characterizes attributes or properties of a subject without using numerical values. It is divided into nominal and ordinal data. Nominal data, as mentioned, categorizes variables into distinct groups without any inherent order, while ordinal data provides a ranking or ordering of these categories based on some criterion. Understanding qualitative data is essential in many research fields, including ophthalmology, as it helps in classifying and analyzing non-numerical attributes such as patient demographics, types of eye diseases, or visual symptoms.

Nominal Data

This is the simplest level of data, which only indicates the name or label of a category.

In ophthalmology, nominal data refers to non-numerical data that categorizes variables without any inherent order or ranking. Here are some examples **(Table 2.2)**.

Ordinal Data

This type of data can be ordered or ranked according to some criterion, but the distance between the values is not meaningful. Examples include satisfaction levels (very unsatisfied, unsatisfied, neutral, satisfied, and very satisfied) and socioeconomic status (low income, medium income, and high income).

TABLE 2.1: Levels of measurements and the power scale.

Nominal	Binary	Ordinal	Discrete	Interval	Ratio
• *Example:* Eye colors • No orderly	• *Gender:* Male or female • *Results:* Pass or fail	• *Examples:* Snellen chart, glaucoma severity scale (GSS) • Ranking	• Countable values • *Example:* No. of patients in the OPD • No. of students in the classroom	• Does not have a true zero point (zero does not indicate the absence of the quantity) • *Example:* Temperature in Celsius or Fahrenheit	• Has a true zero point (zero indicates the absence of the quantity) • *Example:* Height, weight, and age

Basic Concepts and Statistical Tools

TABLE 2.2: Examples of nominal data and some of their characteristics.

Subject/ topic	Examples of nominal data	Explanation
Eye color	"Blue", "green", "brown", "hazel", and "gray"	Colors here are nominal data because they do not have a natural order or ranking
Patient gender	"Male", "female", and "nonbinary"	Patient gender is considered nominal data because it categorizes individuals into groups such as "male", "female", and "nonbinary" without implying any order or ranking
Blood group types	"A", "B", "AB", and "O"	Fall under nominal data because they are used to categorize individuals into different groups without implying any inherent order or ranking
Type of eye disease	"Glaucoma", "cataract", "macular degeneration", and "diabetic retinopathy"	• Nominal classification allows to identify and group these diseases • Grading of severity, response to treatment come later on after this initial categorization
These examples illustrate how nominal data is used to categorize and label variables in ophthalmology without implying any order or hierarchy among the categories. They serve the purpose of classification rather than quantitative measurement		

In ophthalmology, ordinal data refers to data that can be ordered or ranked according to some criterion, but the distances between the values are not meaningful. Here are some examples:

- *Severity of glaucoma:* This can be categorized as mild, moderate, or severe.
- *Visual acuity:* Often measured using categories such as 20/20, 20/40, 20/60, etc., where the order matters but the intervals between them are not consistent.
- *Patient satisfaction:* Categories such as very unsatisfied, unsatisfied, neutral, satisfied, and very satisfied
- *Degree of pain:* Categories such as no pain, mild pain, moderate pain, and severe pain, illustrated in **Figure 2.1**.

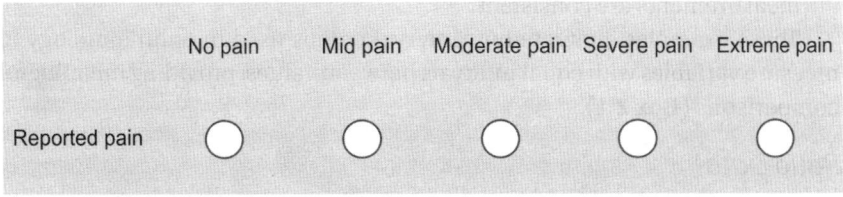

Fig. 2.1: Likert Scale for a typical study to assess Pain Post surgery.

These examples illustrate how ordinal data is used to rank variables in ophthalmology without implying equal intervals between the categories.

Quantitative Data

Quantitative data refers to data that can be measured and expressed numerically, allowing for mathematical and statistical analysis. This type of data is crucial in research and scientific studies as it provides objective information that can be quantified and compared. Quantitative data is broadly categorized into two types—(1) interval data and (2) ratio data. Each type has distinct characteristics that determine how they are used in analysis.

Discrete Data

Discrete data refers to numerical data that can take on only specific, distinct values, and typically countable in nature. These values are often whole numbers with no intermediate values possible. For example, the number of patients visiting an ophthalmology clinic per day, the count of eye surgeries performed, or the number of complications following a procedure. Each of these instances represents separate, countable values that form discrete data sets, allowing researchers to analyze, and draw conclusions based on exact counts and frequencies.

Interval Data

Interval data can be measured on a scale with equal intervals, but the zero point is arbitrary. For example, temperature in Celsius or Fahrenheit. The difference between values is meaningful, but zero does not indicate the absence of the attribute.

In ophthalmology, interval data refers to data that is measured along a scale with equal intervals between values, but without a true zero point. Here are some examples:
- *Intraocular pressure (IOP):* Measurements of IOP, such as 15 mm Hg, 20 mm Hg, and 25 mm Hg, are interval data because the differences between values are consistent.
- *Visual acuity scores:* Scores such as 20/20, 20/40, and 20/60 are interval data as the intervals between the scores are equal.
- *Refractive error measurements:* Values such as –1.00 D, –2.00 D, and –3.00 D for myopia are interval data because the differences between the measurements are consistent.

These examples illustrate how interval data is used in ophthalmology to measure variables with equal intervals between values, providing meaningful comparisons **(Box 2.1)**.

Ratio Data

This type of data can be measured on a scale with equal intervals and a true zero point, which means that zero indicates the absence of the attribute. Examples include age, weight, height, and income. Ratio data allow for a wide range of statistical analyses.

BOX 2.1: Ordinal data versus interval data (AI generated).

When it comes to statistical inferences, both interval and ordinal data have their own unique advantages and applications. However, interval data is generally considered more valuable for statistical inferences due to the following reasons:
- *Equal intervals:* Interval data has equal intervals between values, which allows for a wider range of statistical analyses. This includes calculating means, standard deviations, and performing parametric tests such as t-tests and analysis of variance (ANOVA)
- *More precise measurements:* Interval data provides more precise measurements compared to ordinal data. For example, measurements of intraocular pressure (IOP) in mm Hg or visual acuity scores in logarithm of the minimum angle of resolution (LogMAR) scores like 0.1, 0.2, 0.3, and so on, allow for more detailed and accurate analysis
- *Advanced statistical techniques:* Interval data allows for the use of advanced statistical techniques such as regression analysis, correlation, and factor analysis. These techniques can provide deeper insights into relationships between variables and help in making more accurate predictions
- On the other hand, ordinal data, while useful, has limitations due to the lack of equal intervals between values. This restricts the types of statistical analyses that can be performed

Ordinal data is often used for ranking or categorizing variables, such as severity of glaucoma (mild, moderate, and severe) or patient satisfaction levels (very unsatisfied, unsatisfied, neutral, satisfied, and very satisfied)

In summary, while both types of data have their place in statistical analysis, interval data is generally more valuable for making detailed and accurate statistical inferences

Tabulation of visual acuities and LogMAR notations to indicate the variation in intervals and gaps between the steps

The tabulation of visual acuities and LogMAR notations demonstrates the variation in intervals and discrete steps between each level

In the field of ophthalmology, examples of ratio data include measurements that have a true zero point, allowing for the calculation of meaningful ratios. Some common examples are:
- *Intraocular pressure (IOP):* Measured in millimeters of mercury (mm Hg), IOP is a critical parameter in diagnosing and managing glaucoma. A true zero point indicates the absence of pressure, making it a ratio variable.
- *Corneal thickness:* Measured in micrometers (µm), corneal thickness is essential for assessing corneal health and planning refractive surgeries. The true zero point signifies the absence of corneal tissue.
- *Pupil diameter:* Measured in millimeters (mm), pupil diameter is a vital measurement in evaluating ocular and neurological conditions. A zero value would indicate the absence of a pupil.
- *Axial length:* Measured in mm, axial length refers to the distance from the front to the back of the eye. It is crucial in calculating the power of intraocular lenses for cataract surgery.
- *Retinal thickness:* Measured in µm, retinal thickness is used to assess macular health and detect conditions like macular edema. A zero value represents the absence of retinal tissue.

■ EXAMPLE: VISUAL ACUITY BY SNELLEN VERSUS LOGMAR

Visual acuity is a crucial variable in ophthalmology that measures the clarity or sharpness of vision. It is classified as an ordinal variable because it can be ranked based on levels of vision clarity, such as 20/20, 20/40, and so on. While the values indicate different levels of visual acuity, the intervals between these values are not necessarily equal, and there is no true zero point that represents the complete absence of vision. This *ordinal nature of Snellen visual acuity notation* allows for ranking and comparison of visual acuity among patients, but it does not allow for the calculation of meaningful ratios or the application of interval-based statistics **(Fig. 2.2)**.

Snellen notation is not sufficiently precise for research purposes. Snellen notation, commonly used in clinical settings to measure visual acuity, provides a relative indication of visual clarity, such as 20/20 or 20/40. However, this notation is often insufficient for research purposes due to its lack of precision and inability to capture subtle differences in visual performance.

Visual acuity, often recorded in Snellen notation, is an example of interval data rather than ratio data. While Snellen notation is commonly used in clinical settings to measure and express visual acuity, it does not have a true zero point, making it less powerful for certain statistical analyses.

To enhance the robustness and precision of visual acuity data, especially in research activities, it is to be converted to the LogMAR (logarithm of the minimum angle of resolution) format. This conversion transforms the interval data into a more powerful level that allows for more accurate statistical analysis and comparison. Those values are mentioned in the **Figure 2.2**. The data which represents the order of preferences for example in visual

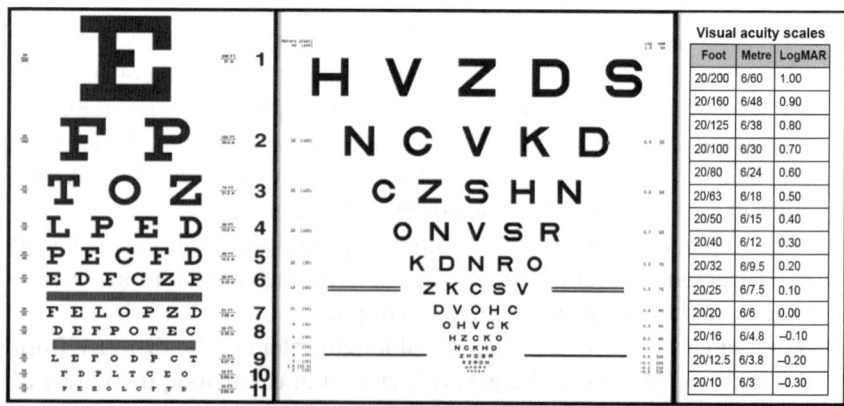

Fig. 2.2: Common in clinical use Snellen chart, LogMAR chart and the equivalence tabulation.
Source: Adapted from Wikipedia. (2025). LogMAR chart [online] Available from https://en.wikipedia.org/wiki/LogMAR_chart [Last accessed March, 2025].

acuity grading, such as 0—no light perception, 1—light perception, 2—hand motion, 3—counting fingers, and so on...

For more detailed and accurate analysis, researchers may rely on other methods, such as LogMAR, which offers a more *granular* measurement of visual acuity, allowing for the detection of smaller changes and a better comparison across different studies. *LogMAR visual acuity notation qualifies as a continuous data.*

By employing visual acuity notations, the LogMAR scales, which give a more uniformly spaced intervals for researchers, one can obtain a more nuanced understanding of the way treatments affect visual acuity; an accurate assessment of effects of disease and treatment modalities are critical for evaluating the effectiveness of treatments, understanding the progression of eye diseases, and developing new interventions. An enhanced precision is particularly important in clinical trials and epidemiological studies, where accurate and reliable data are essential for drawing meaningful conclusions and advancing the field of ophthalmology. It is therefore possible to classify patients in various visual categories in a better manner by using LogMAR visual acuity scaling, as exemplified in the study comparing objective refraction changes after using Nd:YAG laser in treatment of posterior capsular opacification in pseudophakic eyes (A. et al., 2024/06/01) **(Table 2.3)**.

Using Snellen notation in studies may not yield results as robust as LogMAR notation. However, due to study limitations, Snellen acuities are often accepted for publication and addressed during statistical analysis and interpretation. Furthermore, deriving mean or median values from this analysis may be impractical, thereby diminishing the study's

TABLE 2.3: Illustration representing the advantages of BCVA being represented in LogMar from (A et al., 2024/06/01).

Representing BCVA before and after the procedure					
	Mean	*SD*	*Median*	*Percentile 25*	*Percentile 75*
BCVA before procedure	0.3	0.2	0.4	0.2	0.5
BCVA after procedure	0.7	0.2	0.7	0.5	0.8
p-value			<0.001		

BCVA before and after the procedure between ECCE and phacoemulsification groups					
	ECCE		**Phacoemulsification**		
Parameter	*Mean ± SD*	*median (IQR)*	*Mean ± SD*	*median (IQR)*	*p-value*
Preprocedure BCVA	0.16+ .05	0.2 (0.1: 0.2)	0.36 +.014	0.4 (0.3: 0.5)	0.003
Postprocedure BCVA	0.4 + 0.05	0.4 (0.4: 0.5)	0.67 + 0.16	0.7 (0.6: 0.8)	0.003
p-value		0.002			

(BCVA: best-corrected visual acuity; ECCE: extracapsular cataract extraction)
Source: A et al., 2024/06/01.

TABLE 2.4: Representation of Visual Acuities by Snellen Chart and Changes of Visual Acuity being classified by "Improved", "Stayed the same" and "Decreased" (Lei et al., 2024/01/01).

Representation of visual acuities by Snellen chart and changes of visual acuity being classified by "improved", "stayed the same", and "decreased"					
Visual outcomes of patients with pediatric uveitis					
Visual acuity at presentation	Number of patients	Visual acuity at the last follow-up	Number of patients	Change in visual acuity	Number of patients
≤20/200	70/241	≤20/200	19/188	Improved	166/188
(20/200–20/50)	63/241	(20/200–20/50)	30/188	Stayed the same	13/188
>20/50	108/24!	>20/50	139/188	Decreased	9/188

statistical power. Converting Snellen values to LogMAR is often utilized to examine various aspects. However, this approach may introduce inaccuracies due to the differences in how each measurement scales visual acuity and handles variances in testing conditions. Sometimes, therfore the data may be presented without modification and represented in an ordinal variable modality, rather thant continuous variable modality, as illustrated in **(Table 2.4)** from (Lei et al., 2024/01/01). in this approach, howerver, because of the absence of some notations across the continuum, certain nuances and gradations in visual acuity might be lost or misrepresented, leading to potential discrepancies in clinical assessments and research outcomes.

■ CONCLUSION

In conclusion, while Snellen notation has served as a valuable tool in clinical settings, its limitations in precision make it less suitable for research purposes, where more granular data is necessary. The adoption of LogMAR notation, with its continuous data scale, enhances the accuracy of visual acuity measurements, facilitating more reliable statistical analysis and comparisons across studies. By providing a more refined assessment of visual acuity changes, LogMAR notation contributes significantly to the evaluation of treatments and the understanding of eye disease progression, thereby advancing the field of ophthalmology. Moving forward, leveraging LogMAR in research will be instrumental in achieving more robust outcomes and developing innovative therapeutic interventions.

■ BIBLIOGRAPHY

1. Lei B, Zhou X, Gu R, Shu Q, Ding X, Jiang R, et al. Pediatric uveitis in a tertiary referral center in East China: clinical patterns and visual outcomes. J Ophthalmol [Internet]. 2024 (cited 2024/01/01);2024(1):5015614. Available from: https://doi.org/10.1155/joph/5015614
2. Mohamed A, Elagouz M, Mohamed M, Hassan A. Objective refraction changes after using Nd:YAG laser in treatment of posterior capsular opacification in pseudophakic eyes. Egyp J Clin Ophthalmol [Internet]. 2024 (cited 2024/06/01); 7(1):1-8. Available from: https://doi.org/10.21608/ejco.2024.361183

CHAPTER 3

Data Collection Techniques

Nasrin, Bhanu Boddi, Durga Bhavani Mummina

■ INTRODUCTION

In the field of ophthalmology, the precise and methodical collection of data is paramount. Accurate data collection forms the bedrock of informed diagnoses, effective treatment plans, and groundbreaking research. As ophthalmologists, we rely on rigorous data to understand the nuances of eye diseases, the impact of various treatments, and the outcomes of surgeries. This chapter delves into the essential techniques of data collection, tailored specifically for the ophthalmology community. By mastering these techniques, we can enhance our clinical practices, contribute to the advancement of our field, and ultimately, improve patient care.

In the ever-evolving field of ophthalmology, the methods of data collection have expanded to encompass both traditional and modern techniques. The integration of technology has revolutionized how we gather and analyze data, providing deeper insights and more accurate outcomes.

- *Interviews:* These involve directly asking individuals questions to gather information. This method allows for in-depth understanding and clarification of responses.
- *Questionnaires:* Both written and online forms to collect data from respondents are used. Traditional written questionnaires have been complemented by modern online forms, which offer ease of distribution and automated data analysis. These forms can be designed to capture specific patient data, treatment outcomes, and other relevant information.
- *Observations:* These involve watching and recording behaviors or events as they occur. In ophthalmology, this may involve observing patient responses to treatments or documenting the progression of eye conditions over time.
- *Experiments:* These include conducting controlled tests to gather data. This method is essential for clinical trials and research studies aimed at evaluating new treatments or understanding disease mechanisms.

■ DEFINITIONS

Data collection refers to the systematic process of gathering, measuring, and analyzing information from various sources to obtain a comprehensive and accurate understanding of an area of interest. It is a critical step in any research or data-driven decision-making process, ensuring the accuracy and reliability of the results obtained. By employing various methods of data collection, researchers and organizations can effectively gather the necessary data to support their objectives.

Data collection is the process of gathering information from relevant sources to find a solution to a given statistical inquiry. It is the first and foremost step in a statistical investigation. This step is essential because it helps us make informed decisions, identify trends, and measure progress.

■ METHODS OF DATA COLLECTION

Different methods of collecting data include:
- *Interviews:* Directly asking individuals questions to gather information
- *Questionnaires:* Using written or online forms to collect data from respondents
- *Observations:* Watching and recording behaviors or events as they occur
- *Experiments:* Conducting controlled tests to gather data
- *Published sources and unpublished sources:* Using existing data from books, articles, reports, and other documents.

■ STATISTICAL INQUIRY

A statistical inquiry involves an investigation by any agency on a topic where the investigator collects relevant quantitative information. In simple terms, a statistical inquiry is a search for truth using statistical methods of collection, compilation, analysis, interpretation, etc. The basic problem with any statistical inquiry is the collection of facts and figures related to the specific phenomenon being studied. Therefore, the primary purpose of data collection is to gather evidence to reach a sound and clear solution to a problem.

■ TERMS RELATED TO DATA COLLECTION

The terms related to data collection are as follows:
- *Data:* Data serves as a tool that aids an investigator in understanding the problem by providing the necessary information. Data can be classified into two types: Primary data and secondary data.
- *Investigator:* An investigator is the person who conducts the statistical inquiry.
- *Enumerators:* To collect information for a statistical inquiry, an investigator requires assistance from certain individuals known as enumerators.
- *Respondents:* A respondent is an individual from whom the statistical information needed for the inquiry is collected.
- *Survey:* A survey is a method of gathering information from individuals. Its primary purpose is to collect data to describe various characteristics

such as usefulness, quality, price, and kindness. It involves asking questions about a product or service to a large number of people.

■ PRIMARY DATA

Primary data refers to information collected directly from first-hand sources, specifically for a particular research purpose. This type of data is gathered through various methods, including surveys, interviews, experiments, observations, and focus groups. One of the main advantages of primary data is that it provides current, relevant, and specific information tailored to the researcher's needs, offering a high level of accuracy and control over data quality **(Box 3.1 and Table 3.1)**.

Methods of Collecting Primary Data

There are several methods of collecting primary data. Some common methods include:

Interviews

Interviews include collecting data through direct, one-on-one conversations with individuals. The investigator asks questions either directly from the source or from its indirect links.

Direct personal investigation: Involves collecting data personally from the source of origin. For example, directly contacting household women to obtain information about their daily routines.

Illustration: In a study evaluating patient satisfaction post-laser assisted in situ keratomileusis (LASIK) surgery for myopia, a questionnaire was framed

---

BOX 3.1: Sources of data collection.

Primary data collection:
- Direct personal investigation
- Indirect oral investigation
- Information from local sources or correspondents
- *Information through questionnaires and schedules:*
  - Mailed Method
  - Enumerator's method

Secondary data collection:
- Published sources:
  - Government and semigovernment publications
  - Publications of trade associations
  - Journals and papers and international publications
  - Publications of research institutions
- *Unpublished sources*

TABLE 3.1: Illustration of Primary Data being taken from Study and Control group patients (Hervás-Ontiveros, 2024/01/01 #6206).

	Preoperative descriptive statistics of the sample						
	Study group			Control group			
	n	Mean	SD	n	Mean	SD	p value
Preoperative SE (D)	79	0.21	2.84	37	−0.48	4.27	0.187
Preoperative J0 (D)	79	0.04	0.64	37	0.08	0.68	0.380
Preoperative J45 (D)	79	−0.04	0.60	37	0.08	0.54	0.131
IOP (mm Hg)	91	16.63	2.89	69	15.51	2.81	**0.007**
AL (mm)	135	23.27	0.98	141	23.83	1.54	**<0.001**
ACD (mm)	133	3.11	0.49	141	3.26	0.44	**0.005**
K1 (D)	134	43.32	1.70	141	42.97	2.10	0.062
K2 (D)	134	44.39	1.83	141	44.25	2.03	0.269
WTW (mm)	61	11.56	0.81	72	11.72	0.70	0.111
IOL power (D)	145	21.99	2.85	139	20.80	4.03	**0.002**

Note: Bold *p* values indicate statistical significance for the differences between groups. (ACD: anterior chamber depth; AL: axial length; IOL: intraocular lens; IOP: intraocular pressure; K1: flat corneal meridian; K2: steep corneal meridian; SD: standard deviation; SE: spherical equivalent; WTW: white-to-white distance)

and patients' response was recorded pre- and postoperation evaluating their satisfaction.

History was taken about visual complaints from the patients directly in the ophthalmology outpatient department (OPD).

Indirect oral investigation: It involves collecting data orally from someone who has the necessary information, rather than directly from the source. For example, collecting data about employees from their superiors or managers.
- *Advantage:* Provides real-time, natural data; no reliance on self-reported information
- *Disadvantage:* Observer bias, limited to what can be seen, and may influence subjects' behavior
- *Suitable use case:* Behavioral studies and user experience research.

Questionnaires

Questionnaires include collecting data by asking people a set of questions, either online, on paper, or face-to-face. The investigator prepares a questionnaire to collect information, keeping in mind the study's objective.
- *Mailing method:* Involves mailing the questionnaires to informants for data collection, with an attached letter explaining the study's purpose

- *Enumerator's method:* Involves the enumerator personally for reaching out to informants with the prepared questionnaire.
  - *Advantage:* Can reach a large audience quickly and cost-effectively
  - *Disadvantage:* Responses may be biased or inaccurate; low response rates
  - *Suitable use case:* Customer satisfaction surveys and market research.

Illustration: In a study evaluating patient satisfaction post-LASIK surgery for myopia, a questionnaire was framed, and patients' response was recorded pre- and postoperation evaluating their satisfaction.

History is taken about visual complaints from the patients directly in ophthalmology OPD.

Observations

Observations involve collecting data by watching and recording behaviors, events, or conditions as they naturally occur. The observer systematically notes specific aspects of a subject's behavior or the environment, either covertly or overtly.

- *Advantage:* This provides real-time, authentic data without reliance on self-reported information.
- *Disadvantage:* Observer bias can influence the results, and the presence of an observer might alter subjects' behavior.
- *Suitable use case:* Studying user interactions with a product in a natural setting, monitoring wildlife behavior, or assessing classroom dynamics.

Illustration: A study titled "Associations between Retinal and Choroidal Vascularization Parameters and Brachial Artery Flow-mediated Dilation in Type 2 Diabetes and Healthy Controls".

32 eyes of 32 patients were included in this observational study; 15 eyes were categorized into the study group, defined as type 2 diabetic patients without diabetic retinopathy and other diabetic complications, and 17 in the healthy control group. RTVue XR Avanti optical coherent tomography angiography (angio-OCT) was used to perform OCT scans and visualize the superficial and deep retinal plexus [superficial capillary plexus (SCP) and deep capillary plexus (DCP), respectively]. Using OCT image binarization, the choroidal vascularity index (CVI) was calculated. Brachial flow-mediated dilation (FMD) was measured for each participant.

Case–Control Study

In a case–control study, primary data collection involves identifying two groups: Cases (individuals with the condition of interest) and controls (individuals without the condition). Researchers gather data by comparing the exposure to potential risk factors between these two groups.

This method is particularly useful for studying rare diseases or conditions with a long latency period. Researchers meticulously record information about participants' medical history, lifestyle, environmental exposures, and other relevant variables to identify potential associations and causative factors. The strength of this approach lies in its ability to retrospectively analyze data to uncover patterns and potential associations that may inform future research and interventions.

A study aims to analyze the prevalence and severity of posterior capsule opacification (PCO) and glistening in a new hydrophobic biaspheric monofocal intraocular lens (IOLs) 24 months after implantation. In order to verify these parameters and to evaluate material stability during this period, a control group of a well-known and widely studied hydrophobic IOL model was included. All data shown in **Table 3.1** is primary data.

Table 3.1 illustrates primary data being taken from study and control group patients.

Experiments

Experiments involve manipulating one or more variables to determine their effect on another variable within a controlled environment. Researchers create two groups (control and experimental), apply the treatment or variable to the experimental group, and compare the outcomes between the groups.
- *Advantage:* Allows for the establishment of cause-and-effect relationships with high precision.
- *Disadvantage:* Experiments can be artificial, limiting the ability to generalize findings to real-world settings, and they can be resource intensive.
- *Suitable use case:* Testing the efficacy of a new drug, assessing the impact of a new teaching method, or evaluating the effect of a marketing campaign.

Focus Groups

Focus groups involve gathering a small group of people to discuss a specific topic or product, facilitated by a moderator. A group of 6–12 participants engages in a guided discussion led by a moderator who asks open-ended questions to elicit opinions, attitudes, and perceptions.
- *Advantage:* These provide in-depth insights and diverse perspectives through interactive discussions, revealing the reasoning behind participants' thoughts and feelings.
- *Disadvantage:* Results can be influenced by dominant participants or groupthink, and the findings are not easily generalizable due to the small, nonrepresentative sample size.

- *Suitable use case:* Exploring customer attitudes toward a new product, gathering feedback on a marketing campaign, or understanding public opinion on social issues.

Information from Local Sources or Correspondents

Information from local sources or correspondents involves appointing correspondents or local persons at various places to collect data, which is then furnished to the investigator. This method helps cover a wide area.

Illustration: On methods of primary data collection in given in **Box 3.2**.

> **BOX 3.2:** Examples of primary data.
> - *Surveys and questionnaires:* Patients could be asked to complete surveys about their vision quality and any side effects they experience
> - *Interviews:* Researchers might conduct interviews with patients to gather detailed information about their experiences and improvements in vision
> - *Observations:* Clinicians could observe and record changes in patients' vision and eye health over time
> - *Experiments:* The study would involve a controlled experiment where one group of patients receives the new treatment and another group receives a placebo, allowing researchers to compare the outcomes

SECONDARY DATA

Secondary data refers to information that has already been collected, processed, and published by others. This type of data can be sourced from existing research papers, government reports, books, statistical databases, and company records. The advantage of secondary data is that it is readily available and often less expensive to obtain compared to primary data. It saves time and resources since the data collection phase has already been completed **(Boxes 3.1 and 3.2)**.

Sources

Secondary data can be collected through various published and unpublished sources. Here are some examples:

Published Sources

- *Government publications:* These include documents published by the ministries, central, and state governments of India as part of their routine activities. Examples include the Annual Survey of Industries and the Statistical Abstract of India. Government-published statistics are generally reliable.

- *Semigovernment publications:* Semigovernment bodies publish data related to health, education, deaths, and births. Examples include publications from metropolitan councils and municipalities.
- *Publications of trade associations:* Large trade associations collect and publish data from their research and statistical divisions on various trading activities. For example, the Sugar Mills Association publishes data on different sugar mills in India.
- *Journals and papers:* Newspapers and magazines provide a variety of statistical data in their articles, which can be used by investigators for their studies.
- *International publications:* Organizations like the International Monetary Fund (IMF), United Nations organization (UNO), International Labour Organization (ILO), and World Bank publish a variety of statistical information that can be used as secondary data.
- *Publications of research institutions:* Research institutions and universities publish their research activities and findings, which are used by investigators as secondary data. Examples include the National Council of Applied Economics and the Indian Statistical Institute.

Unpublished Sources

Unpublished sources are another means of collecting secondary data. This data is collected by various government and nongovernment organizations for their internal use and is not published. Examples include research work done by professors, professionals, and teachers, as well as records maintained by businesses and private enterprises.

■ CONCLUSION

Both published and unpublished sources serve as vital reservoirs of secondary data that support a wide array of research endeavors. Published sources provide readily accessible and reliable information through government publications, trade associations, international organizations, and research institutions. On the other hand, unpublished sources, often generated for internal use by various entities, offer unique and valuable insights. Together, these sources form the backbone of comprehensive data collection, facilitating informed decision-making and robust academic research.

■ BIBLIOGRAPHY

1. Elsamman A, Mohamed M. Patient satisfaction after laser in situ keratomileusis in myopic patients. Egyp J Clin Ophthalmol [Internet]. 2024 (cited 2024/06/01);7(1):33-41. Available from: https://doi.org/10.21608/ejco.2024.361187

2. Hervás-Ontiveros A, España-Gregori E, Fresno-Cañada C, Butrón-Ruíz R, Cerviño A. Posterior capsular opacification and glistening in hydrophobic monofocal biaspheric intraocular lens two years after implantation: a case control study. J Ophthalmol [Internet]. 2024 (cited 2024/01/01);2024(1). Available from: https://doi.org/10.1155/joph/3520219
3. Małyszczak A, Przeździecka-Dołyk J, Misiuk-Hojło M. Associations between retinal and choroidal vascularization parameters and brachial artery flow-mediated dilation in type 2 diabetes and healthy controls. Open J Ophthalmol [Internet]. 2024 (cited 2024/11/21);18(1). Available from: https://doi.org/10.2174/01187436413398962410110505 21

CHAPTER 4

Sampling Techniques

Krishna Prasad Pallem, B Muniswami

■ INTRODUCTION

Sampling is the process of selecting a subset of individuals from a larger population to represent the whole.

Attempting complete or nearly complete coverage in a statistical study can be costly and time-consuming. Moreover, it may not be necessary to evaluate all or almost all of the population to reach valid conclusions. By studying a sample from the larger population and ensuring that this sample is adequately representative, valid conclusions can be drawn.

There are various methods of sampling, such as random sampling and nonrandom sampling. Under random sampling, one can use simple random sampling, stratified random sampling, systematic random sampling, and cluster random sampling. Each method has its own advantages and applications. Random sampling ensures that every individual has an equal chance of being selected, reducing bias. Stratified sampling involves dividing the population into subgroups and drawing samples from each, enhancing representation across key characteristics. Cluster sampling selects entire groups or clusters, then samples individuals within these clusters to improve efficiency when dealing with large populations. Under nonrandom sampling methods, the sample unit is selected purely based on the discretion of the investigator.

Samples must be chosen carefully to avoid sampling error—when the sample does not accurately reflect the population. Proper design and implementation of sampling techniques are crucial for minimizing errors and biases, which ultimately lead to more reliable and generalizable results. Accurate sampling supports diverse fields such as market research, public health, and social sciences by providing insights into broader trends and behaviors.

While evaluating an entire population might be impractical, well-designed sampling strategies allow researchers to derive meaningful and robust conclusions efficiently.

■ METHODS OF SAMPLING

There are various methods of sampling. The choice of the method will be determined by the purpose of sampling and the nature of the population. The selection of the sample should be done in such a way that the sample taken should be a true representative of the population. There are two ways of taking a sample: One is called random, or probability sampling, and the other is nonrandom sampling.

Random Sampling Methods

Simple Random Sampling with Replacement

This method entails selecting individuals from a population such that each individual is chosen randomly and can be selected more than once. Each draw is independent, meaning the selection of one individual does not influence the selection of another. This approach is particularly useful when dealing with smaller populations or when the same individual might represent different aspects or units of the study.

Random sampling with replacement ensures that the probability of selecting any individual remains constant throughout the sampling process. This method is frequently employed in simulations and probabilistic studies where the variability and independence among samples are crucial.

One advantage of this technique is its ability to provide a truly random and unbiased sample, as each member of the population has an equal chance of being selected multiple times. However, this method can also result in some individuals being selected more than once, which might not be ideal for all types of studies. Despite this, it remains a fundamental technique in the realm of statistics, often serving as a basis for more advanced sampling methods.

Illustration: In ophthalmology, an example of simple random sampling with replacement could involve studying the prevalence of a particular eye condition, such as glaucoma, in a specific population. Researchers might create a database of patients who have had eye examinations within a certain timeframe. Using a random number generator, each patient would be assigned a unique number, and individuals would be selected randomly, with the possibility of being chosen more than once. This method allows researchers to account for variability in the data, ensuring that each patient has an equal chance of being included in the study multiple times. By using this technique, the researchers can gather a truly random and unbiased sample, which can then be analyzed to understand the prevalence and risk factors associated with glaucoma in the population.

Simple Random Sampling without Replacement

This technique involves selecting a subset of individuals from a population in a manner that ensures each individual is chosen randomly and only once. This approach guarantees that each member of the population has an equal chance of being included in the sample, thus providing an unbiased representation of the population. To implement this method, researchers might use random number generators, lottery systems, or other randomization tools.

One notable advantage of simple random sampling without replacement is its ability to minimize duplication and redundancy in the data collected. By ensuring that each individual is selected only once, this method provides a clearer, more accurate picture of the population, enhancing the validity of the study's findings. Furthermore, by avoiding the re-selection of the same individuals, researchers can ensure that their sample is more diverse and representative, capturing a broader range of perspectives and experiences.

Nevertheless, implementing simple random sampling without replacement can be challenging, particularly when dealing with large populations. It requires a comprehensive and up-to-date list of all members of the population, as well as mechanisms to randomize the selection process effectively. Despite these challenges, this method remains a cornerstone of statistical sampling, known for its straightforwardness and reliability.

Illustration: An institution-based cross-sectional study design was conducted on 934 participants who were selected by a simple random sampling method at the entrance of the tertiary eye care and training Center from September to November 2021. A structured questionnaire was used to collect the data through interviews, and the presence or absence, type, and stage of glaucoma were determined by reviewing the chart.

Stratified Random Sampling

When a population is heterogeneous with respect to variables or characteristics under study, stratified random sampling yields better results compared to other sampling methods. This method involves dividing the population into relatively homogeneous groups or strata based on relevant characteristics and then drawing from each group or stratum to produce an overall sample. Each stratum, also known as a subpopulation, ensures representation of all segments of the population or society, such as different areas, classes, and genders **(Fig. 4.1)**.

Systematic Random Sampling

This technique involves selecting every nth individual from a list after a random start point has been established. The process begins by determining the sampling interval (k), which is the ratio of the population size to the desired sample size. For example, if a researcher wants to sample 100 individuals from a population of 1,000, the sampling interval would be 10 ($k = 1000/100$). After every kth individual is selected from the population, and then select.

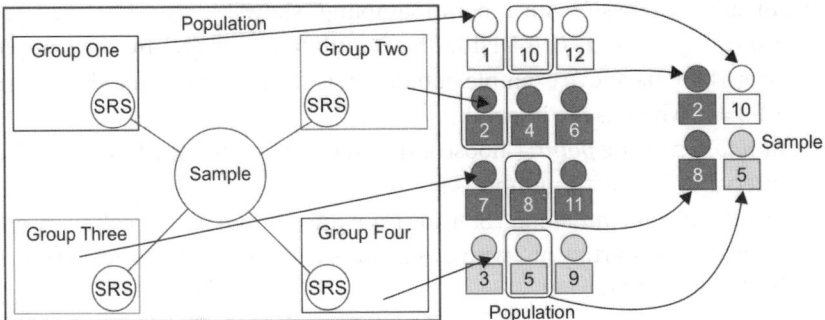

Fig. 4.1: Stratified random sampling.
Source: Adapted from Wikipedia.com. Stratified randomization. [Online] Available from https://en.wikipedia.org/wiki/Stratified_randomization#:~:text=In%20 statistics%2C%20stratified%20randomization%20is,the%20same%20subgroup%20 are%20selected [Last accessed March, 2025].

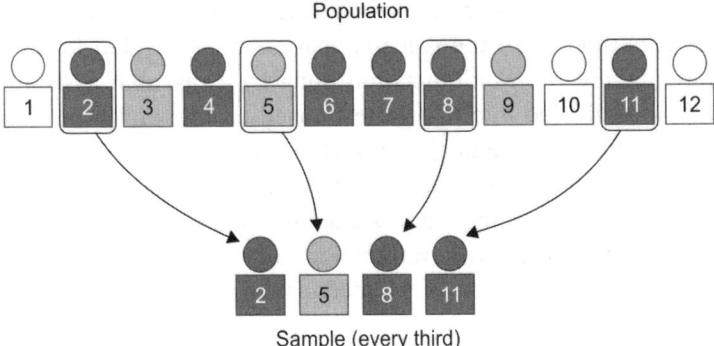

Fig. 4.2: Systematic random sampling.
Source: wikipedia.org. Sampling (statistics). [Online] Available from https://en.wikipedia.org/wiki/Sampling_(statistics)#/media/File:Systematic_sampling.PNG CC BY-SA [Last accessed March, 2025].

Systematic random sampling is efficient and straightforward, particularly useful when dealing with large populations where a simple random sample might be difficult to implement. This method ensures that the sample is spread evenly across the population, reducing the risk of clustering and providing a more accurate representation of the population's diversity. However, it assumes that the list of the population is not ordered in a way that could bias the results **(Fig. 4.2)**.

One advantage of systematic random sampling is its simplicity and ease of implementation. It requires a complete list of the entire population. This makes it a practical choice for situations where compiling a full list might be challenging or time-consuming.

The diagram for "systematic random sampling" shows:
- *Sampling interval (k):* Divide the population size (N) by the sample size(n). In the above example population is 12 and the sample size is 4, so 12/4 = 3, which is the interval.
- *Random starting point:* Choose a starting point within the interval. If the interval is 3, select a number, say 2.
- *Select every nth individual:* Starting from the random point, pick every nth individual. If starting at 2 with 3 as an interval, the chosen individuals will be 2, 5, 8, and 11.

This method ensures systematic, even sampling across the population, enhancing representativeness and diversity.

Illustration: In a study "Effects of music on the preoperative and intraoperative anxiety through the assessment of pupil size and vital signs (blood pressure, respiratory, and pulse rates) among cataract surgery patients at UNTH-Enugu."

Enrolled individuals were randomized into two groups using a systematic sampling method, with the researcher remaining blinded to the group assignments and the randomization done by a research assistant. The patients were divided into two groups based on odd and even numbers, with odd-numbered patients (Group A) receiving surgery with music and even-numbered patients (Group B) undergoing surgery without music, while maintaining sterility with assigned earphones, and their data were meticulously recorded. This randomization was done by the research assistant, and the researcher was blinded to the groups.

Cluster Sampling

In the cluster sampling method, the population is divided into some recognizable subgroups, which are called *clusters*. Now, the random sample of these clusters is drawn, and *all the units* belonging to the *selected clusters* constitute the sample. However, it refers to the sampling procedure, which is carried out in several stages.

Cluster sampling is widely used for geographical studies of many kinds. When the units are spread over a large geographical area, selecting a sampling unit becomes expensive. The area may be divided into convenient subgroups called clusters, select a sample of clusters, and collect the data of all units in each of the selected clusters (**Fig. 4.3**).

For instance, in an ophthalmology study aiming to assess the prevalence of glaucoma in a large region, researchers might employ cluster sampling to efficiently gather data. The region could be divided into numerous smaller geographic areas, or clusters, such as districts and neighborhoods. A random sample of these clusters would then be selected, and all individuals within

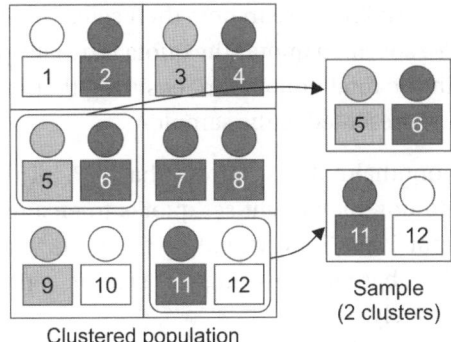

Fig. 4.3: Cluster Sampling illustrated by identifying two clusters.
Source: wikipedia.org. Sampling (statistics). [Online] Available from https://en.wikipedia.org/wiki/Sampling_(statistics)#/media/File:Systematic_sampling.PNG CC BY-SA [Last accessed March, 2025].

the chosen clusters would be examined for glaucoma. This approach would allow researchers to manage resources effectively while still obtaining a representative sample of the larger population.

Nonrandom Sampling Methods

Judgment or Purposive Sampling

Judgment or purposive sampling involves selecting individuals based on the researcher's knowledge and judgment about which participants will be most useful or representative. This method is often used when specific expertise is needed, or when the population of interest is hard to reach or very specific in nature. Researchers rely on their understanding of the study and the population to decide which individuals to include, ensuring that the sample aligns closely with the research objectives. This approach is particularly helpful in qualitative research or exploration studies where an in-depth understanding from a carefully selected group is required.

For instance, in an ophthalmology study investigating a rare eye condition, researchers might use judgment sampling to select participants who have been diagnosed with this rare condition and are receiving specialized treatment. By focusing on these specific individuals, researchers can gather detailed insights and data that might not be available through other sampling methods.

Quota Sampling

Quota sampling is a nonrandom sampling technique where researchers divide the population into exclusive subgroups, as in stratified sampling.

However, in quota sampling, researchers then select individuals from each subgroup based on a specified quota. The quota is usually proportional to the subgroup's share in the total population, ensuring that various segments of the population are represented in the sample.

Illustration: If an ophthalmologist knows that 60% of their patients have myopia and 40% do not, they might set quotas to ensure the study sample reflects these proportions. They would select participants until meeting the quota for each subgroup, ensuring the sample represents the patient demographics accurately.

This method is particularly useful when time and resources are limited, and it allows researchers to ensure diversity in their sample without the need for random selection. However, it is important to note that because the selection within each subgroup is not random, this method may introduce some bias, which should be accounted for when interpreting the results.

Convenience Sampling

Convenience sampling is a nonrandom sampling technique where participants are selected based on their easy availability and proximity to the researcher. This method is often used in exploratory research, pilot studies, or when time and resources are constrained. Convenience sampling can be highly efficient and practical, as it allows researchers to quickly gather data without the need for complex sampling plans. However, it is important to note that this method may introduce significant bias, as the sample may not accurately represent the broader population. As a result, findings from convenience sampling should be interpreted with caution, and researchers should clearly acknowledge the limitations of this approach in their analysis.

Illustration: An ophthalmologist might survey patients in a busy clinic for convenience. However, this method may miss patients who rarely visit the clinic, leading to a nonrepresentative sample. For instance, if the survey aims to study individuals with glaucoma, this approach could overlook those in earlier stages of the disease who do not regularly seek medical attention. These undiagnosed or infrequent visitors might have different characteristics or symptoms compared to the regular patients, resulting in biased findings that do not accurately reflect the entire population affected by glaucoma.

Another example is a medical study examining the effects of a new medication. If researchers select participants from a single clinic where patients are easily accessible, the findings may not be generalizable to patients from diverse geographical areas or different healthcare settings. This convenience sample might introduce bias due to the specific characteristics of the clinic's patient population.

In both cases, convenience sampling offers a practical solution for data collection but requires careful consideration of its limitations and potential biases when interpreting the results.

Snowball Sampling

Snowball sampling is a non-random sampling technique often used when studying hidden or hard-to-reach populations. In this method, the researcher initially contacts a few participants who belong to the population of interest. These initial participants, or "seeds," are then asked to refer to other individuals they know who also belong to the target population. This process continues, "snowballing" into a larger sample as more participants are recruited through referrals.

This technique is particularly useful in research subjects where participants are not easily accessible through conventional sampling methods, such as individuals with rare diseases and marginalized communities.

Illustration: For example, snowball sampling is often employed when researching rare diseases in ophthalmology, such as retinitis pigmentosa. Individuals diagnosed with rare conditions like retinitis pigmentosa, amyotrophic lateral sclerosis, or other uncommon genetic diseases often belong to specific support or community groups. When a patient diagnosed with retinitis pigmentosa visits the hospital, they can be included in the study and informed about it. They are then encouraged to share the study information with other members of their support group.

Snowball sampling can provide valuable insights and access to understudied populations, but it also comes with potential biases, as the sample may become skewed toward individuals within the same social networks. Researchers must acknowledge these limitations and consider them when analyzing and interpreting their findings.

UNIQUE ASPECTS OF SAMPLING TECHNIQUES IN OPHTHALMOLOGY CLINICAL RESEARCH

Sampling techniques in ophthalmology clinical research must address the unique characteristics of the eye and the specific needs of patients with ocular diseases. This paper explores the unique aspects of sampling techniques in ophthalmology clinical research and how they contribute to obtaining reliable and generalizable results.

Specific Considerations in Ophthalmology Sampling

Ophthalmologists must ensure that the sample population accurately represents the diverse patient demographics and ocular conditions encountered in clinical practice. This includes considerations for age, gender, ethnicity, and the prevalence of specific eye diseases in different populations.

Stratified Sampling for Diverse Representations

Stratified sampling is particularly valuable in ophthalmology clinical research, where the prevalence of eye diseases can vary significantly across different demographic groups. By dividing the population into subgroups based on key characteristics such as age, gender, and ethnicity, researchers can ensure that each subgroup is adequately represented in the sample. This enhances the study's ability to draw conclusions that are applicable to a broader population.

Random Sampling for Generalizability

Random sampling remains a cornerstone technique in ophthalmology research, providing an unbiased representation of the population. In studies where the goal is to generalize findings to a larger population, random sampling ensures that every individual has an equal chance of being selected, reducing the risk of bias. This technique is particularly useful in epidemiological studies that aim to understand the prevalence and incidence of eye diseases.

Cluster Sampling for Efficiency

Cluster sampling can be advantageous in ophthalmology clinical research when dealing with large and geographically dispersed populations. By selecting entire clusters, such as community health centers and ophthalmology clinics, and then sampling individuals within these clusters, researchers can efficiently gather data while minimizing logistical challenges. This method is especially useful in multicenter clinical trials and large-scale epidemiological studies.

Addressing Sampling Error and Bias

Accurate sampling is crucial in ophthalmology clinical research to avoid sampling errors and biases that can compromise the validity of the study's findings. Researchers must carefully design and implement sampling strategies to ensure that the sample accurately reflects the population. This involves using appropriate randomization techniques, ensuring adequate sample sizes, and accounting for potential confounding variables.

Minimizing Selection Bias

Selection bias can significantly impact the outcomes of ophthalmology clinical research. To minimize this risk, researchers should use random sampling methods and stratified sampling to ensure that the sample population mirrors the broader population. Additionally, transparent and systematic inclusion and exclusion criteria must be established to avoid overrepresentation or underrepresentation of specific patient groups.

Controlling for Confounding Variables

In ophthalmology research, confounding variables such as comorbid conditions, medication use, and lifestyle factors can influence study outcomes. Researchers must account for these variables in their sampling strategies and data analysis to ensure that their findings accurately reflect the effects of the interventions being studied. This may involve using matched samples, multivariate analysis, and rigorous study design protocols.

Applications of Sampling Techniques in Ophthalmology

Sampling techniques are applied in various ophthalmology clinical research scenarios, including clinical trials, epidemiological studies, and observational research. These techniques enable researchers to investigate the efficacy and safety of new treatments, understand the distribution and determinants of eye diseases, and assess the impact of interventions on patient outcomes.

Clinical Trials

In clinical trials, sampling techniques are used to select participants who meet specific inclusion and exclusion criteria. Random sampling ensures that the trial population is representative of the broader patient population, enhancing the generalizability of the findings. Stratified sampling is often employed to ensure that subgroups of interest, such as patients with different stages of disease, are adequately represented.

Epidemiological Studies

Epidemiological studies in ophthalmology rely on sampling techniques to estimate the prevalence and incidence of eye diseases in different populations. Random sampling and stratified sampling are commonly used to obtain representative samples, while cluster sampling can improve efficiency in large-scale studies. These studies provide valuable insights into the burden of eye diseases and inform public health strategies.

Multistage sampling was used to select 11,786 subjects of all ages from 24 urban clusters and 70 rural clusters in one urban and three rural areas belonging to different parts of Andhra Pradesh, with the aim of obtaining a study sample representative of the urban-rural and socioeconomic distribution of the population of this state.

The Chennai Glaucoma study estimated glaucoma prevalence in Tamil Nadu, India, using population-based sampling with a representative sample.

Stratified sampling was employed by dividing the subjects into subgroups based on age and location to ensure thorough representation. For cluster sampling, 32 villages in rural areas and five clusters in Chennai were selected for data collection.

Observational Research

Observational research in ophthalmology involves studying patient outcomes in real-world settings. Sampling techniques ensure that the study population reflects the diversity of patients seen in clinical practice. Proper sampling allows researchers to draw meaningful conclusions about treatment effectiveness, disease progression, and patient-reported outcomes, ultimately guiding clinical decision-making.

Sampling with Replacement versus Sampling without Replacement

In ophthalmology research, the choice between sampling with replacement and sampling without replacement depends on the study's objectives and design.

Sampling with Replacement

Sampling with replacement is often utilized in simulations and bootstrapping techniques, which are used for estimating the distribution of a statistic. This method is particularly useful when the sample size is small, and researchers need to create multiple resamples to assess the variability of their findings. For example, in genetic studies of eye diseases, sampling with replacement can help in estimating the genetic diversity within a small population.

Sampling without Replacement

Sampling without replacement is more commonly applied in clinical trials, epidemiological studies, and observational research. This method ensures that once a participant or data point is selected, it is not chosen again, which is crucial for maintaining the integrity and independence of the sample. For instance, in a clinical trial evaluating a new treatment for glaucoma, sampling without replacement ensures that each patient receives the treatment only once, preventing duplication and bias in the results. Similarly, in large-scale epidemiological studies, sampling without replacement helps in accurately estimating the prevalence of eye diseases by ensuring that the same individuals are not counted multiple times.

By understanding when to use sampling with replacement versus sampling without replacement, ophthalmology researchers can better design their studies to achieve reliable and valid results.

■ CONCLUSION

Sampling techniques in ophthalmology clinical research are essential for obtaining reliable and generalizable results. By carefully designing and implementing sampling strategies that account for the unique characteristics of the eye and patient populations, researchers can minimize errors and biases, leading to more accurate and impactful findings. These techniques support the advancement of ophthalmology by providing robust evidence that informs clinical practice, public health policies, and the development of new treatments.

■ BIBLIOGRAPHY

1. Ezepue CO, Anyatonwu OP, Duru CC, Odini F, Nwachukwu NZ, Onoh C, et al. Frontiers | Effects of music on the preoperative and intraoperative anxiety through the assessment of pupil size and vital signs (blood pressure, respiratory, and pulse rates) among cataract surgery patients at UNTH-Enugu. Front Ophthalmol [Internet]. 2024 (cited 2024/01/15);3. Available from: https://doi.org/10.3389/fopht.2023.1340752
2. George R, Arvind H, Baskaran M, Ramesh SV, Raju P, Vijaya L. The Chennai glaucoma study: Prevalence and risk factors for glaucoma in cataract operated eyes in urban Chennai. Indian J Ophthalmol [Internet]. 2010 (cited May-Jun 2010);58(3):243-5. Available from: https://doi.org/10.4103/0301-4738.62655
3. Kovai V, Krishnaiah S, Shamanna BR, Thomas R, Rao GN. Barriers to accessing eye care services among visually impaired populations in rural Andhra Pradesh, South India. Indian J Ophthalmol [Internet]. 2007 (cited 2007 Sep-Oct);55(5):365-71. Available from: https://doi.org/10.4103/0301-4738.33823
4. Yekunoamelak BZ, Ayele FA, Bogale ZM, Worku EM. Frontiers | Proportion and associated factors of glaucoma among outpatient department at university of Gondar comprehensive specialized hospital tertiary eye care and training center, northwest Ethiopia, 2021. Front Ophthalmol [Internet]. 2025 (cited 2025/03/05);5. Available from: https://doi.org/10.3389/fopht.2025.1521263

CHAPTER 5

Charts and Graphs

Sunil Moreker, Keerthana Bonsi, B Punyavathi

■ INTRODUCTION

This chapter explores essential tools and graphs for data analysis in medical research. It covers various charts and their importance in presenting complex information clearly. Understanding these tools aids in interpreting and communicating scientific findings effectively. The following sections detail graphical methods such as bar graphs and boxplots, crucial for visualizing data trends and patterns.

Bar graphs are instrumental in comparing categorical data, allowing researchers to easily discern differences among groups. For instance, a bar graph could compare the prevalence of different diseases across various age groups. Boxplots, on the other hand, are useful for summarizing data distributions and identifying outliers. They provide insights into the spread and skewness of the data, which is vital for understanding variability within a dataset.

The chapter will also discuss line graphs, which are particularly useful for examining changes over time. In medical research, a line graph might depict the progression of patient recovery rates throughout a clinical trial. Scatter plots will be explored as well; they can illustrate relationships between two variables, such as the correlation between physical activity and blood pressure levels.

Furthermore, we will delve into more advanced techniques, such as heat maps, which can display large volumes of data by using color coding to represent values. This method is especially helpful in genetic research where patterns within vast datasets need to be identified.

By mastering these tools, researchers can enhance their ability to analyze and present data effectively, leading to more precise conclusions and informed decisions in the field of medical research.

■ BAR GRAPHS

Bar charts are utilized to compare various categories of data. Each bar denotes a specific category, with its height or length corresponding to the value associated with that category. Bar charts can be displayed either vertically or horizontally, allowing flexibility in presentation depending on the nature of the data. They are particularly effective for displaying discrete data and making quick comparisons between different groups. Variations of bar charts include stacked bar charts, which show multiple data series within a single bar, and grouped bar charts, where bars representing different categories are placed next to each other for easy comparison. The clarity and simplicity of bar charts make them a popular choice for visualizing categorical data in fields such as business, education, and research as illustrated in **(Fig. 5.1)** for a study on average foraminal stenosis grades in patients with idiopathic Horner's Syndrome by Ong, et al. (2025).

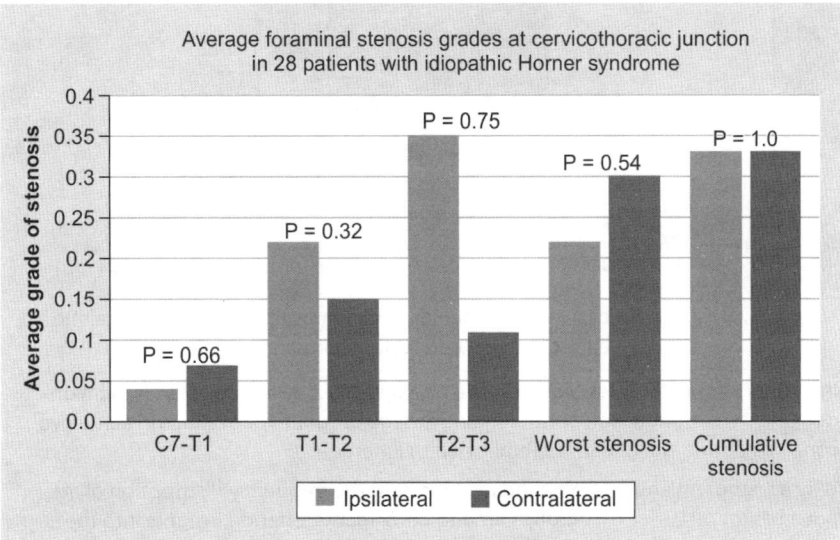

Fig. 5.1: Bar diagram showing the average grade of foraminal stenosis between the C7 and T2 segments of the spine in patients with Horner syndrome.

This bar graph from Ong, et al. (2025) represents an investigation of the etiopathogenetic factors of otherwise seemingly idiopathic Horner syndrome caused by cervicothoracic foraminal stenosis between the C7 and T3 segments	
Relevance of bar diagrams in such situations	• In the study of idiopathic Horner syndrome caused by cervicothoracic foraminal stenosis between the C7 and T3 segments, bar diagrams are crucial • They illustrate comparative data of stenosis, highlighting differences in average grades and aiding in identifying patterns linked to the syndrome. This visual simplification allows for quick analysis and clear communication of findings

■ HISTOGRAMS

These are similar to bar graphs but are used to represent the distribution of a single variable. The data is divided into bins, and the height of each bar represents the frequency of data points within each bin as illustrated in (**Fig. 5.2**) for participants in an online Ophthalmic emergency related support program from (Townsend et al., 2025/01/14).

Illustration

The illustration is given in **Figure 5.2**.

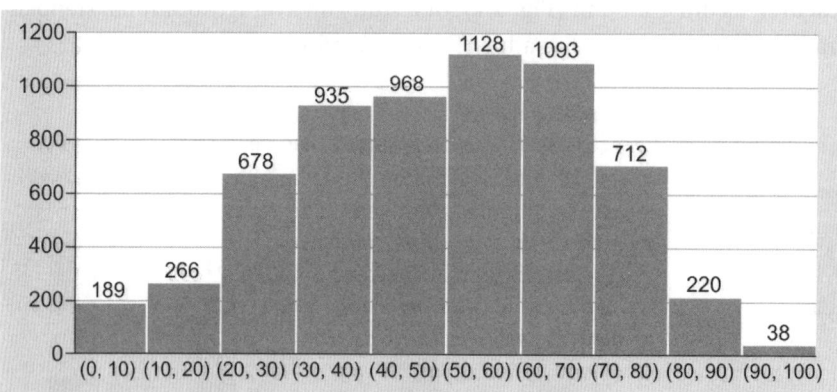

Fig. 5.2: Histogram depicting the age of participants in an online ophthalmic emergency-related support program.

In a study aiming to determine baseline demographics and usage trends of an on-demand, synchronous teleophthalmology triage program for evaluating acute eye concerns during the COVID-19 Public Health Emergency	
Why a histogram and not a bar graph?	• Histograms represent the frequency distribution of age groups among participants, offering insights into the distribution pattern. Unlike bar graphs, which compare categories, histograms focus on a single variable, making them ideal for understanding age demographics in the study • The median age of patients was 51 (interquartile range, 36–65) years • If the data was normally distributed then mean ($\mu \pm \sigma$) would have been a better indicator of central tendency; but since this data is not normally distributed hence median is better representor of central tendency (M_d)

▪ PIE CHARTS

These are circular charts divided into sectors, each representing a proportion of the whole. They effectively show the relative sizes of parts compared to the entire entity.

Pie charts are commonly used in business, media, and other fields to display data visually and make complex information easier to understand. Each sector, or "slice," corresponds to a category's percentage of the total.

The size of each slice is proportional to its contribution to the whole, making it straightforward to compare different categories.

For instance, in a pie chart representing market shares of various companies, a larger slice indicates a higher market share. Pie charts are particularly useful when showing the composition of a dataset where the total sum is meaningful, such as budget allocations, survey results, or population demographics.

The utility of pie chart is well illustrated by the represeatation of various categories for Prevalence of PCO grading in the control Group sample and study group samples in **Figure 5.3** by (Hervás-Ontiveros et al., 2024/01/01).

However, pie charts can be less effective when there are too many categories or when the differences between categories are very small, as it may become difficult to differentiate the slices. In these cases, alternative visualizations such as bar charts or histograms might be more appropriate **(Fig. 5.3)**.

Illustration

The illustration is given in **Figure 5.3**.

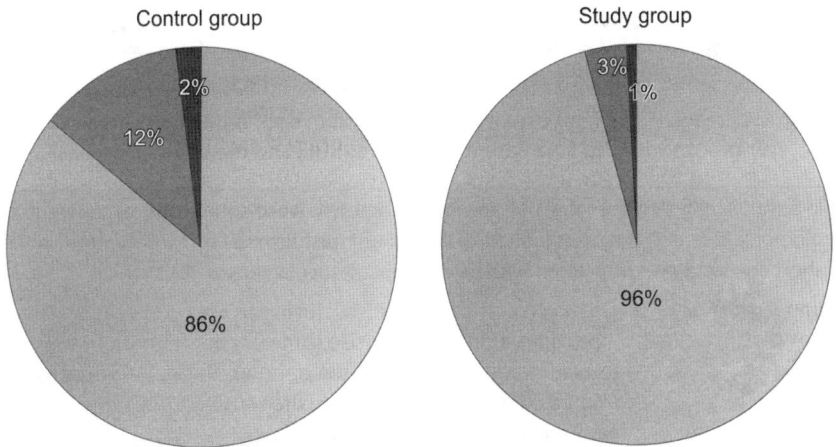

Fig. 5.3: Pie chart to present sizes of various subgroups.

In a study analyzing the prevalence and severity of posterior capsule opacification (PCO) and glistening in new hydrophobic biospheric monofocal intraocular lenses (IOLs)	
It is important to represent the two groups with internal subgroups	Pie charts are preferable in scenarios where you want to show the relative proportions of different groups that make up a whole. They provide an intuitive visual representation, making it easy to see the contribution of each part at a glance

■ BOXPLOTS

They summarize data by providing key statistics such as the median, which is the value separating the higher half from the lower half of the data set. They also show the interquartile range (IQR), which measures the spread of the middle 50% of the data, and identify outliers, which are data points that fall significantly outside the typical range of the data. The box plot is illustrated in **(Fig. 5.4)** from article by (Rementería-Capelo et al., 2025/01/01) on biometry of short and long eyes groups with both the Barrett universal II (BUII) and the Barrett true axial.

Illustration

The illustration is given in **Figure 5.4**.

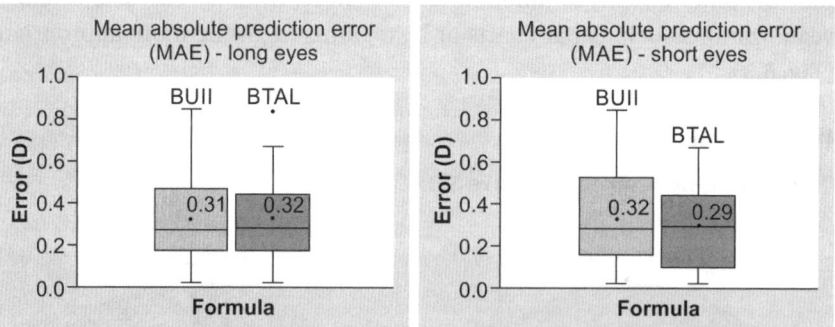

Fig. 5.4: Image Depicting boxplot of "Mean absolute error (MAE) for short and long eyes groups with both the Barrett universal II (BUII) and the Barrett true axial".

In a study analyzing the refractive accuracy of a novel swept-source optical coherence biometer (SS-OCT) that uses individual refractive indices to measure axial length, in short and long eyes implanted with monofocal intraocular lenses (IOLs)	
Importance of box plot	• The box plot is particularly useful in this context because it provides a clear and concise summary of the central tendency and dispersion of the data, which can be crucial for understanding the refractive accuracy using SSOCT in eyes with short and long axial lengths • Unlike bar graphs that focus on comparing categorical data, or Bland-Altman plots that assess agreement between measurement methods, box plots can highlight the variability within each group reveal the presence of *outliers*, and show the interquartile range which represents the middle 50% of the data. This level of detail is vital for clinical studies where understanding the spread and consistency of measurements can impact the interpretation of the results and subsequent clinical decisions

■ LINE GRAPHS

These are used to display data points connected by straight lines. They are particularly useful for showing trends over time, as illustrated by **(Fig. 5.5)** from study of Post surgical IOP controls in phacoemulsification (Control) with phacoemulsification combined with micro bypass stent (Tsao et al., 2024/01/01).

Illustration

The illustration is given in **Figure 5.5**.

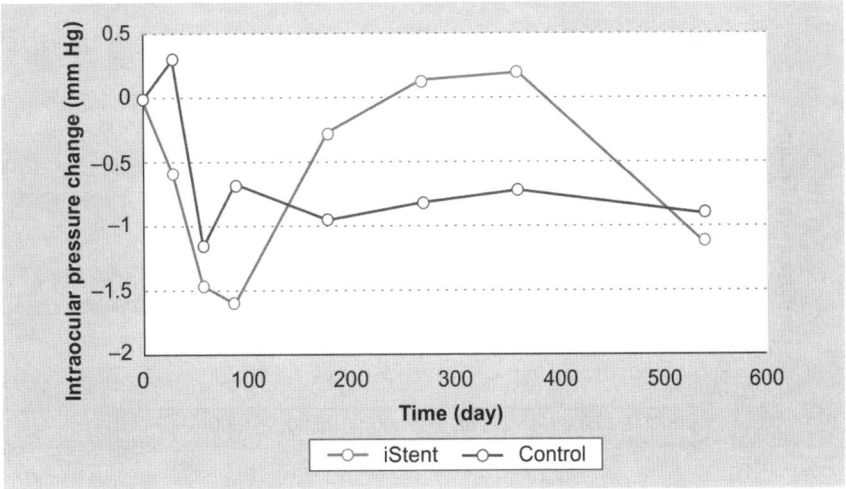

Fig. 5.5: Postsurgical IOP controls in phacoemulsification (Control) with phacoemulsification combined with a micro-bypass stent.

The study by Tsao et al. (2024) compared intraocular pressure (IOP) control postphacoemulsification alone versus phacoemulsification combined with micro-bypass stent. It was evident that open-angle glaucoma or normotensive glaucoma patients benefitted better with combined surgery reducing the need to use postsurgery antiglaucoma medications to keep IOP in a normal range	
Importance of line chart in the above context	Line graphs are crucial in this context as they allow for the clear visualization of IOP trends over time postsurgery in the two groups, control postphacoemulsification alone versus phacoemulsification combined with a micro-bypass stent. By connecting data points with straight lines, line graphs make it evident how combined surgery offers superior benefits in glaucoma patients, reducing the need for postsurgery antiglaucoma medications

■ SCATTER PLOTS

These plots use dots to display the values of two different variables. They are practical for identifying relationships or correlations between variables.

For example, in a scatter plot, each point represents an observation with coordinates corresponding to its values on the two variables being compared. This visual representation makes it easier to see patterns, trends, and possible outliers within the data.

Scatter plots are commonly used in fields such as statistics, economics, and social sciences to analyze and interpret data, helping researchers understand how one variable may affect or relate to another.

Axial length and spherical equivalen relations ship are reperesented well by use of Scatter Plots **(Fig. 5.6)** (A. et al., 2024/06/01).

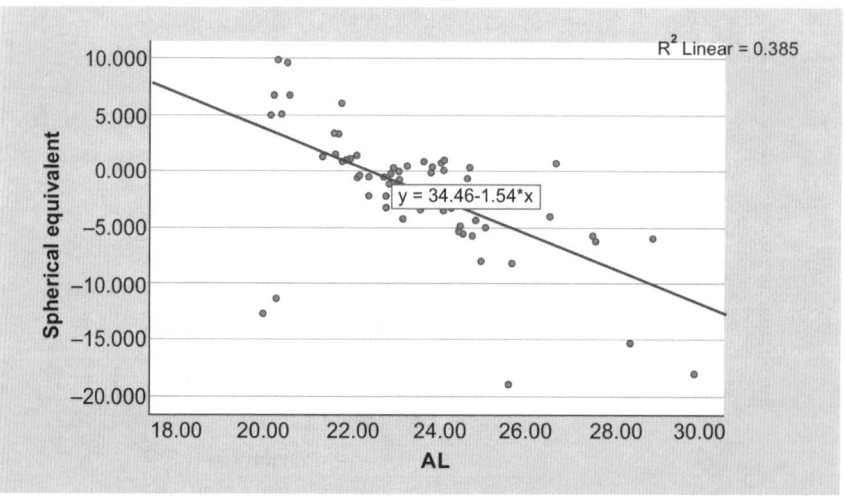

Fig. 5.6: Scatter plots of the axial length and the spherical equivalent.

This is from a study investigating the effect of axial length and spherical equivalent (SE) on the peripapillary retinal nerve fiber layer (RNFL) and ganglion cell complex (GCC)	
Why scatter plot is relevant to this situation	• Scatter plots are ideal for showing the relationship between axial length, spherical equivalent, RNFL, and GCC. By plotting these variables, patterns and correlations become clear. The figure used shows a significant moderate positive correlation between SE and the RNFL average, including the superior and inferior quadrants • Alternatively, a line graph can also be used to illustrate trends and relationships between these variables over time or across different conditions • In this example, there is a highly significant moderate positive correlation between SE and RNFL average, RNFL superior quadrant, and RNFL inferior quadrant as correlation coefficient (r) = (0.43, 0.56, and 0.42, respectively) and p value (<0.0001, <0.0001, and <0.0001, respectively) as shown in this table. A Simple linear regression analysis was calculated to predict RNFL thicknesses based on SE. A significant regression equation was found

In conclusion, selecting the appropriate chart or graph is crucial for effectively conveying data insights. Pie charts are valuable for illustrating the proportions of different groups within a whole, providing an intuitive visual representation of relative contributions. Scatter plots, on the other hand, are excellent for demonstrating relationships or correlations between two variables, as evidenced by the study investigating the effect of axial length and spherical equivalent on the RNFL and GCC. This study found significant moderate positive correlations, highlighted by specific correlation coefficients and p values. Additionally, line graphs can be employed to depict trends and relationships over time or across various conditions, offering another layer of data visualization. Ultimately, the choice of visual representation depends on the nature of the data and the specific insights one aims to communicate.

■ BLAND ALTMAN PLOT

These are used to assess the agreement between two different measurement methods. They plot the differences between the measurements on the y-axis against the averages of the measurements on the x-axis. The plots include lines for the mean difference (bias) and the limits of agreement (typically the mean difference ± 1.96 times the standard deviation of the differences). This helps to identify any systematic bias and the range within which most differences between the methods lie.

Bland-Altman plots are used to compare the Toric IOL related measurements taken by two different devices to illustrate aong with the confidence limits Axis estimates (Yang et al., 2024/01/01) **(Fig. 5.7)**.

■ FOREST PLOT

Forest plots are graphical representations used in meta-analyses to display the relative strength of treatments in several studies. In the context of a noninferiority trial, a forest plot helps illustrate that the new treatment is not worse than the standard treatment by more than a prespecified margin. Each line in the plot represents a study, with a central marker indicating the effect estimate and horizontal lines, representing confidence intervals Forest plot usage is illustrated in the study of systemic antimicrobials with placebo by (Sridharan & Sivaramakrishnan, 2017/11/22) **(Fig. 5.8)**.

■ HEAT MAPS

Heat maps are a versatile tool in ophthalmology that provides a visual representation of variations across a surface or within a volume. In topography, heat maps are used to display the curvature of the cornea, allowing for the detection of irregularities such as astigmatism or keratoconus. These maps,

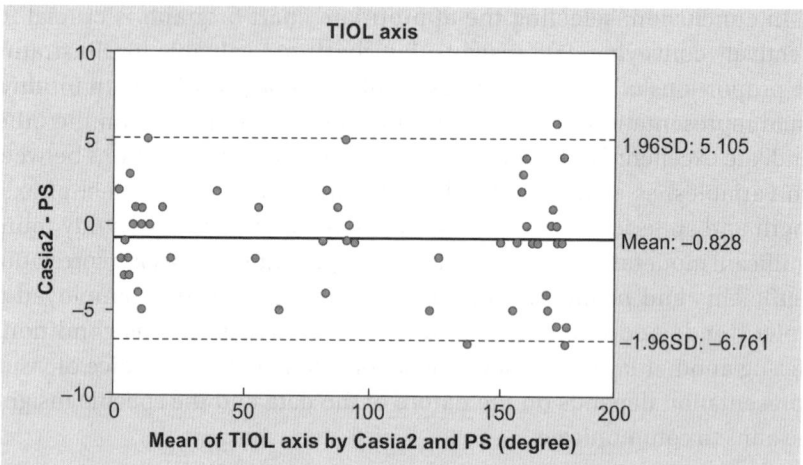

Fig. 5.7: Bland-Altman plot applied to illustrate the confidence limits in Toric IOL-related axis estimates.

This graphic presents the comparative accuracy and reliability of postoperative toric intraocular lens (TIOL) alignment measurement by 2 methods: Casia2 and Adobe Photoshop with digital slit lamp images (PS method)	
Advantages of the Blan-Altman plots	• Bland-Altman plots are advantageous for evaluating the agreement between two measurement methods. They visualize systematic bias by plotting the mean difference and limits of agreement, making them simple, interpretable, and versatile. These plots offer detailed insights into the relationship between methods, highlighting any proportional bias and ensuring a comprehensive understanding of comparative accuracy • The study by Yang et al. (2024) demonstrated that Casia2 and PS exhibited a high level of agreement in measuring postoperative TIOL alignment, as indicated by the intraclass correlation coefficient (ICC) analysis ($ICC_{2,1}$ 0.999) and Bland–Altman plot (mean difference −0.828°). Although the 95% level of acceptability (LoA) appears broad (−6.761° to 5.105°), rotations under 10° typically result in <0.50 D of astigmatism, which may not be clinically significant

as shown in **Figure 5.9**, provide detailed color-coded images that highlight areas of steep or flat curvature, facilitating diagnosis and treatment planning.

In corneal topography, heat maps are used to visualize the curvature of the cornea, allowing for the detection of irregularities such as astigmatism or keratoconus. By representing different curvatures with varying colors, heat maps enable clinicians to easily identify areas of steep or flat curvature and track changes over time. This is particularly useful in diagnosing and

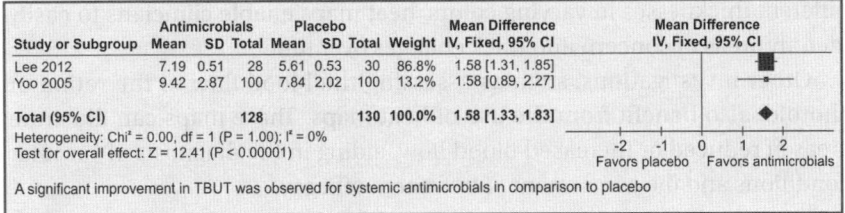

Fig. 5.8: Representing forest plot of test of systemic antimicrobials with placebo.

Explanation for the above **Figure 5.8**, representing forest plot of TBUT of systemic antimicrobials with placebo.

In a study titled "Therapies for Meibomian Gland Dysfunction: A Systematic Review and Meta-Analysis of Randomized Controlled Trials"

Importance of forest plot	• Forest plots are graphical representations used in meta-analyses to display the relative strength of treatments in several studies • Depicts the pooled analysis of TBUT of two systemic antimicrobials (one each with minocycline and doxycycline) with placebo and was favoring the antimicrobials with an MD of 1.58 [1.33, 1.83]

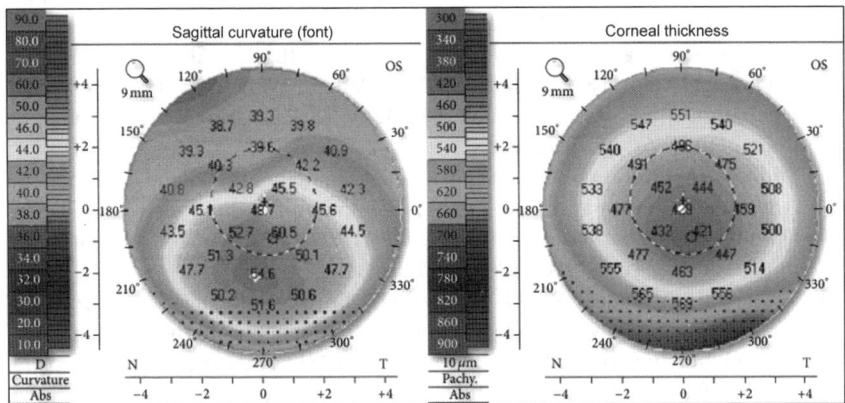

Fig. 5.9: The colors accompanying the central image with mapping of the keratometry values give the diagnostic cues.
Source: https://en.wikipedia.org/wiki/File:Corneal_topography,_stage_II_keratoconus_(Elise_A._Slim_et_al.).svg CC BY.

monitoring corneal conditions, planning refractive surgeries, and fitting contact lenses.

Similarly, in optical coherence tomography (OCT) scans, heat maps are employed to visualize the retinal layers' thickness and any variations therein. This is particularly useful in diagnosing and monitoring conditions such as macular degeneration, diabetic retinopathy, and glaucoma. By representing different thicknesses in varying colors, heat maps enable clinicians to easily identify areas of concern and track changes over time.

Other investigations, such as assessing the blood flow in the retina or choroid, also benefit from the use of heat maps. These maps can illustrate areas of reduced or increased blood flow, aiding in the diagnosis of vascular conditions and the assessment of treatment efficacy.

■ BIBLIOGRAPHY

1. Hervás-Ontiveros A, España-Gregori E, Fresno-Cañada C, Butrón-Ruíz R, Cerviño A. Posterior Capsular Opacification and Glistening in Hydrophobic Monofocal Biaspheric Intraocular Lens Two Years After Implantation: A Case Control Study. J Ophthalmol [Internet]. 2024 (cited 2024/01/01);2024(1). Available from: https://doi.org/10.1155/joph/3520219
2. Mustafa A, Mostafa E, Mounir A, Mostafa A. Effect of axial length on pripapillary retinal nerve fibre layer (RNFL) using optical coherence tomography (OCT). Egypt J Clin Ophthalmol [Internet]. 2024 (cited 2024/06/01);7(1):43-53. Available from: https://doi.org/10.21608/ejco.2024.361188
3. Ong J, Kurokawa M, Khanna S, De Lott LB, Kurokawa R, Sharma A. Frontiers | Computed tomography-based investigation of degenerative neural cervicothoracic foraminal stenosis as a potential mechanism for Horner syndrome. Front Ophthalmol [Internet]. 2025 (cited 2025/01/07);4. Available from: https://doi.org/10.3389/fopht.2024.1497845
4. Rementería-Capelo LA, Contreras I, García-Pérez JL, Ruiz-Alcocer J. Refractive Accuracy of a Novel Swept-Source OCT in Patients With Short and Long Eyes. J Ophthalmol [Internet]. 2025 (cited 2025/01/01);2025(1). Available from: https://doi.org/10.1155/joph/9987580
5. Sridharan K, Sivaramakrishnan G. Therapies for Meibomian Gland Dysfunction: A Systematic Review and Meta-Analysis of Randomized Controlled Trials. Open Ophthalmol J [Internet]. 2017 (cited 2017/11/22);11(1):346-54. Available from: https://doi.org/10.2174/1874364101711010346
6. Townsend NA, Shah S, Reyes J, Townsend JH, Bozung A, Ricur G, et al. Frontiers | Tele-ophthalmology as an effective triaging tool for acute ophthalmic concerns. Front Ophthalmol [Internet]. 2025 (cited 2025/01/14);4. Available from: https://doi.org/10.3389/fopht.2024.1511378
7. Tsao Y-T, Yeh P-H, Su W-W. Comparison of Phacoemulsification Alone and With Trabecular Microbypass Stent in Primary Open-Angle Glaucoma and Normal-Tension Glaucoma. J Ophthalmol [Internet]. 2024 (cited 2024/01/01);2024(1). Available from: https://doi.org/10.1155/2024/4034215
8. Yang B, Lai C, Qin Y, Lin H, Wang S, Liao H, et al. Pilot Study on Postoperative Toric Intraocular Lens Alignment. J Ophthalmol [Internet]. 2024 (cited 2024/01/01);2024(1). Available from: https://doi.org/10.1155/2024/1053914

CHAPTER 6

Measures of Central Tendency

Nasrin, Jaya Siresha Nakka, Durga Bhavani Mummina

■ INTRODUCTION

Although frequency distributions serve useful purposes, there are many situations that require other types of data summarization. Measures of central tendency are sometimes needed to make meaningful interpretations of the data. Generally, it is found that in any distribution, values of the variables tend to congregate around the central value of the distribution. This tendency of the distribution is known as its central tendency and the measures devised to consider this tendency are known as measures of central tendency.

In statistical terms, a distribution refers to the way in which values of a variable are spread or dispersed across a range. It represents the frequencies of different outcomes or values observed in a dataset and can take various shapes, such as normal, skewed, or uniform distributions. Understanding the distribution of data is crucial for selecting appropriate measures of central tendency and for making accurate interpretations and decisions based on the data.

The most common measure of central tendency is the arithmetic mean, often simply referred to as the "mean" or "average." The arithmetic mean is computed by summing all the values in a data set and dividing by the number of values, providing a single value around which the data points tend to cluster. As such, in many contexts, the terms "average" and "arithmetic mean" are used interchangeably to denote this measure of central tendency.

■ ARITHMETIC MEAN/AVERAGE

In common parlance, the terms "arithmetic mean" and "average" are often used interchangeably and refer to the same concept. Both represent a central value around which the data points tend to cluster, providing a simple and intuitive summary of the dataset **(Figs. 6.1 and 6.3)**.

Ungrouped Data

Definition

The mean, often referred to as the average, is the sum of all values in a data set divided by the number of values **[Tables 6.1(a) and 6.1(b)]**.

$$\text{Mean } (\bar{X}) = \frac{1}{n}\sum_{i=1}^{n} x_i$$

Measures of Central Tendency

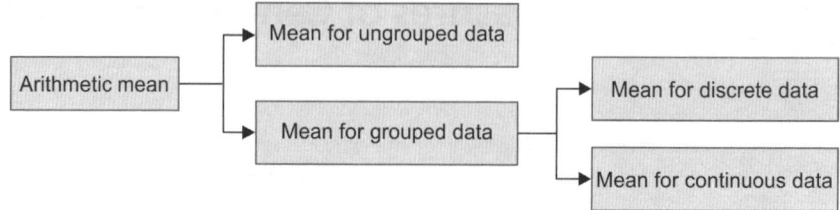

Fig. 6.1: Classification of arithmetic mean.

Illustration

Ungrouped data are illustrated in **Tables 6.1(a) and 6.1(b)** (Gh. et al., 2024/12/01).

TABLE 6.1(a): Representation of age of study participants as ungrouped data (Gh. et al., 2024/12/01).

Baseline data of the 30 studied participants with MPSs		
Baseline data	N = 30	
Age (years)		
Mean ± SD	9.40 ± 2.76	
Median (range)	9 (5–14)	
Sex, n (%)		
Male	19	(63.3)
Female	11	(36.7)

TABLE 6.1(b): Explanation for illustration of ungrouped data from (Gh. et al., 2024/12/01).

In the study "Ophthalmic Manifestations in Patients with Mucopolysaccharidosis Attending Assiut University Children Hospital"	
Ungrouped data versus grouped data	Ungrouped data is a simple representation of data without any further grouping or classification in the above example; the age of study participants has simply been represented as mean ± standard deviation (SD) without any further grouping

Grouped Data

Mean for Discrete Data

Definition: The mean for discrete data is calculated by taking the sum of all the individual data values and dividing it by the total number of data values. This provides the central tendency of the data set by giving an average value.

$$\text{Mean}(\bar{x}) = \frac{\Sigma fx}{n}$$

Illustration

This is illustrated in **Tables 6.2(a) and 6.2(b)** from (A. et al., 2024/06/01).

TABLE 6.2(a): Illustration of mean for grouped data: Short, medium, and long eyes based on axial length (A. et al., 2024/06/01).

GCC thickness measurements based on axial length (AL) groups				
	Axial length groups			
Measurements	AL <21 8	AL 21–24 31	AL >24 30	*p* value
Ganglion cell complex (GCC) average thickness: Mean ± SD Median (range)	100.3 ± 5.5 100.5 (92–108)	100 ± 10.4 101 (9–128)	96.8 ± 5 97 (84–107)	0.09
Post hoc tests	P1 = 0.99, P2 = 0.52, P3 = 0.26			
GCC superior mean ± SD Median (range)	99.6 ± 5.9 99 (92–109)	100 ± 13.6 99 (81–154)	96.9 ± 5.7 97.5 (83–109)	0.5
Post hoc tests	P1 = 0.99, P2 = 0.77, P3 = 0.42			
GCC inferior: Mean ± SD Median (range)	101 ± 6 103.5 (92–108)	100 ± 9.4 102 (76–126)	96.4 ± 5.4 96.5 (84–107)	0.03*
Post hoc tests	P1 =0.09, P2 = 0.046, P3 = 0.02			
P1 = AL <21 vs. AL 21–24; P2 = AL <21 vs. AL >24; P3 = AL21–24 vs. AL >24				

TABLE 6.2(b): Explanation for illustration from (A. et al., 2024/06/01).

In the study on the effect of axial length on the peripapillary retinal nerve fiber layer (RNFL) using optical coherence tomography (OCT)	
Grouped data versus ungrouped data	• For grouped data, patients would be categorized based on predefined ranges of axial lengths (e.g., short, medium, and long eyes) • This categorization helps in simplifying the data collection process and ensures consistency in data interpretation

Continuous Data

Calculate the arithmetic mean of patients suffering from eye diseases from the below age-related classification in a month **(Table 6.3).**

$$\bar{x} = A + \frac{1}{N} \Sigma_{i=1}^{n} f_i d_i$$

Illustration

The illustration is provided in **Table 6.3** from (A et al. 2022/12/01).

Properties of Arithmetic Mean

- Algebraic sum of deviations set of values from their arithmetic mean is "zero". If x_i/f_i, $i = 1, 2, 3,....n$ is the frequency distribution, then $\Sigma_{i=1}^{n} f_i(x_i - \bar{x}) = 0$, $\bar{x}$ is being the mean of the distribution.

TABLE 6.3: Continuous data for the visual acuity at baseline and follow-up from (A et al. 2022/12/01).

Baseline and follow-up visual acuity	
Descriptive variables	**Number of patients**
Baseline visual acuity:	
6/60	1 (6.3%)
6/18	1 (6.3%)
Hand motion	6 (37.5%)
PL with good projection	2 (12.5%)
PL with bad projection	5 (31.3%)
No perception of light	1 (6.3%)
Follow-up visual acuity:	
6/60	1 (6.3%)
6/36	1 (6.3%)
6/18	1 (6.3%)
2/60	2 (12.5%)
1/60	3 (18.8%)
0.50/60	1 (6.3%)
Hand motion	2 (12.5%)
Good perception of light	4 (25%)
No perception of light	1 (6.3%)
Visual acuity (by logmar):	
Baseline	2.83 ± 0.70
Follow-up	1.93 ± 0.84
p-value	<0.001

Visual acuity by logMAR having a mean for continuous data

Data expressed as frequency (percentage) and mean (SD). p-value was significant if <0.05.

- The sum of the squares of the deviations of a set of values is minimum when taken about mean.
- *Mean of composite series:* If $\bar{x}_i$ ($i = 1, 2,....k$) are the means of k component series of sizes n_i ($i = 1, 2,...k$) respectively, then the mean $\bar{x}_i$ of the composite series obtained on combining the component series is given by the formula:

$$\bar{x}_i = \frac{\sum (n_i\, x_i)}{\sum n_i}$$

Merits and Demerits of Arithmetic Mean

Merits:
- *Simplicity:* The arithmetic mean is easy to calculate and understand.
- *Comprehensive:* It considers all data points in the dataset, providing a complete summary.
- *Mathematical properties:* It has useful mathematical properties, making it suitable for further statistical analysis.
- *Central tendency:* It provides a measure of central tendency, indicating the average value of the dataset.
- *Consistency:* It is consistent and reproducible, meaning the same dataset will always yield the same mean.

Demerits:
- *Sensitivity to outliers:* The arithmetic mean is highly sensitive to extreme values (outliers), which can distort the result.
- *Not always representative:* In skewed distributions, the mean may not accurately represent the central tendency.
- *Not suitable for all data types:* It is not appropriate for ordinal or nominal data, as it requires numerical values.
- *Affected by sample size:* In small samples, the mean can be less reliable and more influenced by individual data points.
- *Misleading in heterogeneous data:* In datasets with high variability, the mean may not provide a meaningful summary.

■ MEDIAN/CENTRAL VALUE

To put it in simpler terms, the median can indeed be referred to as the "central value" of a dataset. This is because it represents the point at which half the values are below and half are above, making it a valuable measure when dealing with skewed distributions. Unlike the arithmetic mean, the median is not influenced by extreme values or outliers, providing a more resilient central tendency measure in such cases (**Figs. 6.2 and 6.3**).

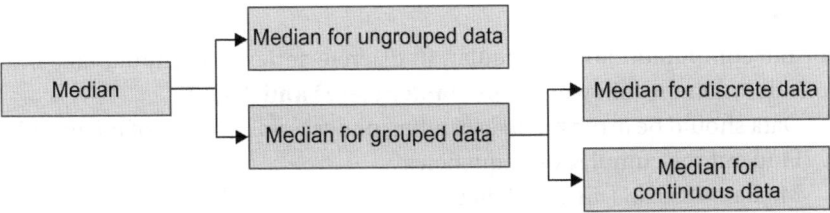

Fig. 6.2: Classification of median.
Source: Sankar Foundation Data Base.

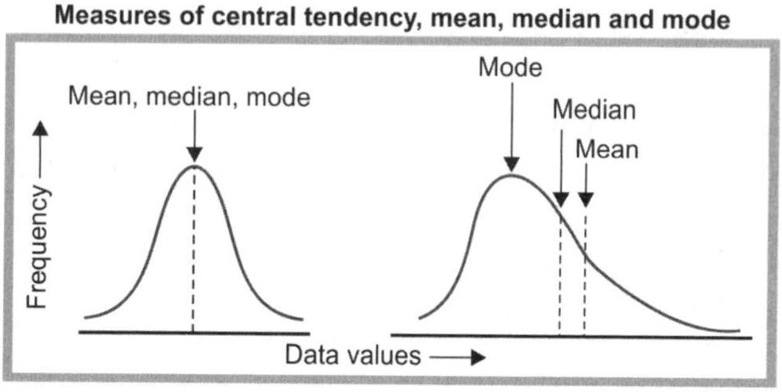

Fig. 6.3: Mean, median, and mode for the normally distributed data and mean, median, and mode for the skewed data.

Ungrouped Data

Definition

The median is the middle value in a data set when the values are arranged in ascending or descending order. If the number of values is even, the median is the average of the two middle numbers.

- If (n) is odd: Median = $\dfrac{(n+1)\text{th}}{2}$ observation
- If (n) is even:
  - Arrange the data in ascending order.
  - Identify the two middle values.
  - Calculate the average of these two middle values.
  - The formula for the median when n is even is:

$$\text{Median} = \dfrac{x_{\frac{n}{2}} + x_{\frac{n}{2}+1}}{2}$$

Illustration

Odd data:
For the data set [3, 5, 7, 9, 11]: Median = 7

Even data:
For the data set [3, 5, 7, 9]
Median = (5 + 7)/2 = 6

Grouped Data

For the computation of the median in discrete series, one should take into consideration the following steps [**Tables 6.4(a) and 6.4(b)**]:
1. Data should be arranged in ascending or descending order of magnitude.
2. Find out the cumulative frequencies.
3. Median = size of $(n+1)/2$th item
4. Find out the value of $(n+1)/2$ or the next higher to this and then determine the value corresponding to it. This will be the value of median.

Measures of Central Tendency

Illustration

Illustration for mean and medin in grouped data is provided in **Table 6.4(a)** from (A et al. 2024/06/01)

TABLE 6.4(a): Mean and median for the grouped data (A et al. 2024/06/01).

GCC thickness measurements based on axial length (AL) groups				
	Axial length groups			
Measurements	AL<21 8	AL 21–24 31	AL >24 30	p value
GCC average thickness: Mean ± SD Median (range)	100.3 ± 5.5 100.5 (92–108)	100 ± 10.4 101 (9–128)	96.8 ± 5 97 (84–107)	0.09
Post hoc tests	P1= 0.99, P2 = 0.52, P3 = 0.26			
GCC superior mean ± SD Median (range)	99.6 ± 5.9 99 (92–109)	100 ± 13.6 99 (81–154)	96.9 ± 5.7 97.5 (83–109)	0.5
Post hoc tests	P1 = 0.99, P2 = 0.77, P3 = 0.42			
GCC inferior: Mean ±SD Median (range)	101 ± 6 103.5 (92–108)	100 ± 9.4 102 (76–126)	96.4 ± 5.4 96.5 (84–107)	0.03*
Post hoc tests	P1 = 0.09, P2 = 0.046, P3 = 0.02			
P1 = AL <21 vs. AL 21–24; P2 = AL <21 vs. AL > 24; P3 = AL21–24 vs. AL >24				

TABLE 6.4(b): Explanation for illustration of mean and median in grouped data in **Table 6.4(a)**.

Effect of axial length on peripapillary retinal nerve fibre layer (RNFL) using optical coherence tomography (OCT)	
Median for discrete data	In the above example, the median for discrete data that is ganglionic cell thickness for different axial lengths divided into three groups has been represented

Continuous Data

The median for continuous data involves a slightly different approach than for discrete data. The computation is as follows [**Tables 6.5(a) and 6.5(b)**]:
- Arrange the data in ascending order.
- Determine the class interval containing the median. This is identified by finding the cumulative frequency just greater than $(n + 1)/2$.

The formula to calculate the median for continuous data is given by:

$$\text{Median} = L + \left(\frac{\frac{n}{2} - C_f}{f} \right) \times h$$

Measures of Central Tendency

The mean and median in situations for continuous data is illustrated well by the Visual acuity representations by Logmar in [___ / Chap ___]. In additions the differential blood parameters provided in **Table 6.5(a)** from (Guttmann et al., 2025/02/27) for study categories based on onset of symptoms and are described below.

	Differential blood parameters in COVID-19 patients.							
	With new-onset ocular symptoms				Without new-onset ocular symptoms			
	n	Median	Min	Max	n	Median	Min	Max	p value
Lymphocytes (in %)	25	30	4	48.8	130	26	10	59	0.239
C-reactive protein (in mg/dL)	25	9.1	0.1	51	130	9.47	0.1	64.12	0.643
Interleukin-6 (in pg/mL)	11	49.1	2.2	3,190	34	111	11.5	4,980	0.277
Ferritin (in ng/mL)	19	1,044.37	72	11,424.9	93	1,113.88	40.32	15,452	0.503
D-dimers (in µg/L)	13	1,310	330	64,568	71	1,393.00	302	54,500	0.940

Blood parameters are compared in terms of number, median, minimum, and maximum values between patients with new-onset ocular symptoms and those without. Additionally, the *p* values (determined through the Mann-Whitney U test) are reported

TABLE 6.5(b): Explanation for illustration from (Guttmann et al., 2025/02/27 in **Table 6.5(a)**.

Ocular symptoms in COVID-19 patients with a history of hospitalization in the first pandemic wave in Styria, Austria	
Why median in this situation?	• The data set is possibly not following a normal distribution (must be mentioned elsewhere in the literature). Therefore, the median is a more appropriate measure of central tendency • In cases where the data is skewed or contains outliers, the mean can be heavily influenced by extreme values and may not accurately reflect the central location of the data. The median, on the other hand, represents the middle value when the data is ordered and is less affected by outliers and skewness

Properties of Median

- *Central tendency:* The median is a measure of central tendency, representing the middle value in a data set when the values are arranged in ascending or descending order.

- *Robustness:* The median is less affected by outliers and skewed data compared to the mean. This makes it a more robust measure of central tendency in such cases.
- *Positional measure:* The median is a positional measure, meaning it depends on the position of values in the data set rather than their magnitude.
- *Uniqueness:* For a given data set, the median is unique. There is only one median value for any set of numbers.
- *Data requirement:* The median can be calculated for ordinal, interval, and ratio data, but not for nominal data.
- *Even and odd data sets:*
  - For an odd number of observations, the median is the middle value.
  - For an even number of observations, the median is the average of the two middle values.
- *Divides data:* The median divides the data set into two equal halves, with 50% of the values below it and 50% above it.
- *Nonadditive:* Unlike the mean, the median is not additive. This means the median of the combined data sets is not necessarily the sum of the medians of the individual data sets.

Merits and Demerits of Median

Merits:
- *Not affected by outliers:* The median is not influenced by extremely high or low values, making it a reliable measure for skewed distributions
- *Simple to calculate:* It is straightforward to compute, especially for small datasets.
- *Representative of the middle:* The median represents the middle value, providing a clear indication of the central tendency.
- *Useful for ordinal data:* It can be used with ordinal data, where the mean cannot be applied.
- *Graphical representation:* The median can be easily located on a cumulative frequency graph.

Demerits:
- *Ignores extreme values:* While this can be an advantage, it also means that the median does not consider all data points, potentially missing important information.
- *Not suitable for further statistical analysis:* Unlike the mean, the median cannot be used for further algebraic calculations.
- *Less sensitive to data changes:* Small changes in the dataset may not affect the median, which can sometimes make it less responsive to variations in the data.

- *Interpolation required:* In continuous data, finding the exact median may require interpolation.
- *Not always unique:* For even-numbered datasets, the median is the average of the two middle numbers, which may not be an actual data point.

■ MODE/COMMON VALUE

In common parlance, the mode can indeed be referred to as the "common value" because it represents the most frequently occurring number in a data set. However, it is not typically called an "average value" because "average" usually refers to the mean in everyday language. The mode is particularly useful in understanding the most typical value in a data set, especially when dealing with categorical data or data with repeated values **(Fig. 6.3)**.

Ungrouped Data

The mode is the value that appears most frequently in a data set. A data set may have one mode, more than one mode, or no mode at all.

Illustration

For the data set [1, 2, 2, 3, 4]: Mode = 2
For the data set [1, 1, 2, 2, 3]: Mode = 1 and 2 (bimodal).

Illustration

The mode of visual acuity is the most frequently occurring score in the data set. If the visual acuity score of 80 appears more frequently than any other value in this group, then:

$$Mode = 80$$

This indicates that the visual acuity score of 80 is the most common measurement among the patients.

Grouped Data

The mode is the value that appears most frequently in a data set.

The mode is useful for discrete data to identify the most common value. This aids fields such as healthcare by highlighting prevalent conditions or symptoms, aiding in resource allocation and treatment planning.

[**Tables 6.6(a) and 6.6(b)**] illustrates, how an ophthalmology clinic can tabulate data for prioritizion of care and management patient flow based on common symptoms. We have data on the number of patients visiting an ophthalmology clinic for different types of eye conditions over a month. The data is grouped into different classes based on the number of visits.

TABLE 6.6(a): Depicting frequency of ophthalmic symptoms in patients visiting the ophthalmology clinic during a conjunctivitis epidemic.

Name of the symptom	Frequency during normal season	Frequency during conjunctivitis epidemic season
Tearing	5	35
Pain	12	10
Redness	18	25
Loss of vision	9	8
Other	6	8

TABLE 6.6(b): Explanation for **Table 6.6(a)**, depicting frequency of symptoms.

In a departmental audit data, the tabulation depicting the frequency of ophthalmic symptoms in patients visiting the ophthalmology clinic during a conjunctivitis epidemic shows applicability of the mode (unpublished data)	
The benefits of mode compared to mean and median	• The mode is useful for nominal data and skewed distributions because it is not affected by outliers. In a conjunctivitis epidemic, it highlights common symptoms for better resource allocation • Unlike the mean and median, the mode is straightforward, reflecting what is typical in a dataset, making it valuable in medical statistics and retail

Continuous Data

In a continuous series, the modal class should be ascertained first. Mode is defined as the value having maximum frequency. In another way by preparing the grouping and analysis, mode is calculated by applying the following formula:

$$\text{Mode} = L + \frac{(f_1 - f_0)}{2f_1 - f_0 - f_2} \times h$$

Suppose we have the data representing the intraocular pressure (IOP) (in mm Hg) of a group of cataract patients posted for surgery as in **Table 6.7**:

The modal class is 16–18, since it has the highest frequency of 15.
L = 16
h = 2 is the width of the class interval
f_1 = 15
f_0 = 12 = frequency of the class preceding the modal class
f_2 = 10 = frequency of the class succeeding the modal class

TABLE 6.7: Representing intraocular pressure (IOP) and frequency to illustrate mode.

IOP range (mm Hg)	Frequency (patients)
10–12	5
12–14	8
14–16	12
16–18	15
18–20	10
20–22	6

Properties of Mode

The mode has several important properties that make it a valuable measure of central tendency:

- *Simplicity:* The mode is easy to understand and calculate. It simply identifies the most frequently occurring value in a dataset, offering a straightforward measure of central tendency.
- *Applicability to categorical data:* The mode is the only measure of central tendency that can be used with nominal data (categorical data), such as colors, types, or categories. This makes it versatile for various types of data analysis.
- *Unaffected by extreme values*: Unlike the mean, the mode is not affected by extremely high or low values (outliers) in the dataset. This makes it a robust measure of central tendency in skewed distributions.
- *Relevance to real-world scenarios:* The mode often represents the most typical or common value in a dataset, which can be very useful in practical situations. For example, in market research, the mode can indicate the most preferred product or service.
- *Multiple modes:* A dataset can have more than one mode (bimodal or multimodal), which provides additional insights into the distribution of the data. However, this property can also be a demerit as it might complicate interpretation.
- *Nonnumeric data:* The mode can be used with nonnumeric data, making it versatile for various types of data analysis. This flexibility is particularly useful when dealing with qualitative data.

Merits and Demerits of Mode

Merits:

- *Simplicity:* The mode is easy to understand and calculate. It simply identifies the most frequently occurring value in a dataset.
- *Applicability to categorical data:* The mode is the only measure of central tendency that can be used with nominal data (categorical data), such as colors, types, or categories.

- *Unaffected by extreme values:* Unlike the mean, the mode is not affected by extremely high or low values (outliers) in the dataset. This makes it a robust measure of central tendency in skewed distributions.
- *Relevance to real-world scenarios:* The mode often represents the most typical or common value in a dataset, which can be very useful in practical situations. For example, in market research, the mode can indicate the most preferred product or service.
- *Multiple modes:* A dataset can have more than one mode (bimodal or multimodal), which provides additional insights into the distribution of the data.
- *Nonnumeric data:* The mode can be used with nonnumeric data, making it versatile for various types of data analysis.

Demerits:
- *Not always unique:* A dataset can have more than one mode (bimodal or multimodal), which can make interpretation difficult. In some cases, there may be no mode at all if no value repeats.
- *Not suitable for small datasets:* In small datasets, the mode may not provide a meaningful measure of central tendency, as it can be heavily influenced by minor variations.
- *Ignores data distribution:* The mode only considers the most frequent value and ignores the rest of the data distribution. This can lead to a loss of information about the overall dataset.
- *Less stable:* The mode can be less stable than the mean or median, especially in datasets with a large number of unique values. Small changes in the data can result in a different mode.
- *Limited use with continuous data:* For continuous data, the mode is less useful because it requires grouping data into intervals, which can be arbitrary and affect the result.
- *Not always representative:* The mode may not always represent the central tendency of the data, especially in skewed distributions or when the most frequent value is an outlier.

■ GEOMETRIC MEAN

The geometric mean, sometimes called the "central multiplier" or "multiplicative average," is a way to find an average that is more suitable for data involving growth rates, ratios, or proportional comparisons. It is particularly useful when the values are multiplied together or are exponentially related, giving a better central value than simply adding them up.

For example, in ophthalmology, the geometric mean can be used to analyze visual acuity measurements across different populations. If you have a set of visual acuity scores that vary widely, using the geometric mean can provide a more accurate representation of the central tendency, helping to better understand the overall visual performance of the group.

Another example is in the study of optical aberrations, such as astigmatism. The geometric mean can be used to analyze and average the refractive errors across different meridians of the eye. This helps in understanding and correcting vision problems more accurately.

Geometric means are a measure of central tendency that indicates the central value of a set of numbers by using the product of their values. It is particularly useful for sets of numbers whose values are meant to be multiplied together or are exponentially related.

$$GM = \sqrt[n]{a_1 \times a_2 \times a_3 \times \ldots \times a_4}$$

Illustrations

- *Chromatic adaptation:* The geometric mean is used in models of chromatic adaptation, which is the ability of the human visual system to adjust to changes in lighting conditions to maintain consistent color perception. A weighted geometric mean (WGM) method has been proposed to improve the prediction of sensory and cognitive adaptation in human observers
- *Optical aberrations:* In the study of optical aberrations, such as astigmatism, the geometric mean can be used to analyze and average the refractive errors across different meridians of the eye. This helps in understanding and correcting vision problems more accurately
- *Visual acuity measurements:* When comparing visual acuity measurements across different populations or conditions, the geometric mean can provide a more accurate representation of central tendency, especially when the data is skewed or has a wide range of values.

■ HARMONIC MEAN

The harmonic mean is a type of average that is particularly useful when dealing with rates or ratios. Unlike the arithmetic mean, which is calculated by simply adding up the values and dividing by the number of values, the harmonic mean takes the reciprocals of the values, finds their arithmetic mean, and then takes the reciprocal of that result.

To put it in other words, the harmonic mean is especially handy when you need to average things such as speeds, rates, or ratios. It gives more weight to smaller values, which can be very useful in certain medical and scientific contexts.

When evaluating surgical videos, such as those analyzing cataract surgeries, the harmonic mean can be used to improve the detection of pupil reactions. By calculating the harmonic mean of recall, precision, and ground truth coverage rate (GTCR), the software can more accurately segment and track the pupil and iris sizes throughout the video. This enhances the quality of surgical assessments and outcomes.

In the automated identification of phases in cataract surgery videos, the harmonic mean is used to calculate the Dice score. This score is the harmonic mean of precision and recall (sensitivity) and helps in the precise detection of the pupil boundary. By using the harmonic mean, the assessment becomes more reliable, ensuring better results in machine learning models.

The harmonic mean is a powerful tool for averaging rates and ratios, providing a more accurate central tendency in specific contexts. For ophthalmologists, its applications in surgical video analysis and machine learning can greatly enhance the accuracy and reliability of various assessments. Understanding and utilizing the harmonic mean in your practice can lead to improved outcomes and better patient care.

The harmonic mean is another measure of central tendency, which is calculated as the reciprocal of the arithmetic mean of the reciprocals of a set of numbers. It is particularly useful in situations where the average of rates or ratios is desired.

$$HM = \frac{n}{\frac{1}{x_1} + \frac{1}{x_2} + \ldots + \frac{1}{x_n}}$$

Illustrations

In the field of ophthalmology, as illustrated in surgical video analysis software programs, the harmonic mean is used in various contexts. For example, in the evaluation of surgical videos, the harmonic mean of recall, precision, and GTCR is used to detect pupil reactions in cataract surgery videos.

This helps in improving the quality of surgeries by providing accurate segmentation and tracking of the pupil and iris sizes across the entire video.

Additionally, the harmonic mean is used in the assessment of automated identification of phases in videos of cataract surgery using machine learning and deep learning techniques.

This involves calculating the Dice score, which is the harmonic mean of precision and recall (sensitivity), for the detection of the pupil boundary.

■ CONCLUSION

In summary, the harmonic mean plays a crucial role in the field of ophthalmology, particularly in the analysis of surgical videos and the implementation of machine learning models. Its ability to provide a more reliable measure of central tendency for rates and ratios ensures higher accuracy and improved outcomes in the detection and segmentation of critical features during cataract surgeries. By integrating the harmonic mean into their practices, ophthalmologists can enhance the quality of patient care and surgical precision.

■ BIBLIOGRAPHY

1. ElSedfy Gh, Tohamy D, Mahmoud H, Bakr SH, Khalaf SH. Ophthalmic manifestations in patients with mucopolysacc-haridosis attending assiut university children hospital. Egypt J Clin Ophthalmol [Internet]. 2024 (cited 2024/12/01);7(2). Available from: https://doi.org/10.21608/ejco.2024.404127
2. Guttmann A, Heidinger A, Woltsche N, Brodmann M, Kurzmann-Gütl K, Nemecz V, et al. Frontiers | Ocular symptoms in COVID-19 patients with a history of hospitalization in the first pandemic wave in Styria, Austria. Front Ophthalmol [Internet]. 2025 (cited 2025/02/27);5. Available from: https://doi.org/10.3389/fopht.2025.1540904
3. Hamza A, Abd El-Rahman M, Ali T, El-Sebaity D. Corneal collagen crosslinking for the treatment of microbial keratitis. Egypt J Clin Ophthalmol [Internet]. 2022 (cited 2022/12/01);5(2):67-77. Available from: https://doi.org/10.21608/ejco.2022.280969
4. Mustafa A, Mostafa E, Mounir A, Mostafa A. Effect of axial length on pripapillary retinal nerve fibre layer (RNFL) using optical coherence tomography (OCT). Egypt J Clin Ophthalmol [Internet]. 2024 (cited 2024/06/01);7(1):43-53. Available from: https://doi.org/10.21608/ejco.2024.361188

CHAPTER 7

Measures of Dispersion

Suparna G, B Punyavathi

■ INTRODUCTION

Understanding the distribution and variability of data is fundamental in statistical analysis. Measures of dispersion play a crucial role in this process, offering insight into the spread and consistency of data points within a dataset. These measures provide a deeper comprehension of the data's behavior, beyond central tendency metrics such as the mean or median. By quantifying the extent to which data points differ from one another, measures of dispersion help identify patterns, outliers, and the overall reliability of the data.

Measures of dispersion include a variety of statistical tools, each with its unique characteristics and applications. Some of the most common measures include the range, variance, standard deviation, and interquartile range (IQR). Each measure offers a different perspective on data variability, and selecting the appropriate measure depends on the nature of the data and the specific analysis goals.

The range, as the simplest measure of dispersion, provides a quick assessment of data spread by identifying the difference between the maximum and minimum values. However, it is susceptible to outliers and may not accurately reflect the overall distribution of data points. On the other hand, the variance and standard deviation, which consider the squared differences between each data point and the mean, offer a more comprehensive view of data variability but require more complex calculations.

The IQR represents the middle 50% of data points by measuring the difference between the first (25th percentile) and the third quartile (75th percentile). This measure is particularly useful for identifying the spread of the central portion of the dataset while mitigating the influence of outliers. Understanding these measures of dispersion enables researchers and analysts to make more informed decisions, enhance data interpretation, and improve the quality of statistical analyses.

■ RANGE

The range is a measure of dispersion that indicates the spread of data points in a dataset. It is one of the simplest measures of variability and is defined as the difference between the maximum and minimum values in the dataset. The formula for calculating the range is:

$$Range = Maximum\ value - Minimum\ value$$

The range provides a quick sense of the extent of variability in the data **(Tables 7.1 and 7.2)**.

However, it is sensitive to outliers, as it only considers the extreme values and ignores the distribution of the rest of the data points. Despite this limitation, the range is useful in various contexts, such as:
- *Initial data analysis:* The range can be used as a preliminary measure to understand the spread of the data before applying more complex statistical analyses.
- *Quality control:* In manufacturing and quality control processes, the range is often used to monitor the consistency of product measurements.
- *Comparative studies:* The range can be used to compare the variability of different datasets, especially when the datasets have similar sizes and distributions.

Illustration

Among 14 patients who received anti-VEGF injections for ARMD, it was found that the total number of injections received per person was mentioned in **Table 7.1**.

TABLE 7.1: Data on number onf injectins received by each patient.														
Patient index no.	1	2	3	4	5	6	7	8	9	10	11	12	13	14
Number of injections received	1	5	3	1	2	2	7	12	8	3	4	7	5	5
Comments: Average number of injections received by patients (mean): 4.64 Minimum values: 1; maximum values: 12; 25 percentile: 2.25; 75 percentile: 6.5; 50th percentile (median): 4.5; Commonest (mode): 5														

The range of the distribution depicted in **Table 7.1** will be 12 – 1.

$$\text{Range} = \text{Maximum value} - \text{Minimum value}$$
$$= 12 - 1 = 11.$$

While the range is easy to compute and understand, it has limitations, such as being sensitive to extreme values or outliers. Therefore, it is often used alongside other measures of central tendency and variability, like the mean, median, and standard deviation, to give a more comprehensive picture of the data's distribution.

Handling outliers effectively is essential in statistical analysis as they can skew results. The process involves identifying outliers using methods like the Z-score or IQR (outside the scope of this book), examining their causes, deciding whether to remove, transform, or use robust statistical methods,

Measures of Dispersion

and documenting every step for transparency. This ensures more accurate and reliable data analysis.

TABLE 7.2: Example of a series of 14 diabetic retinopathy patients receiving multiple doses of anti-VEGF injections No. of injections received over a period of 3 years follow-up (unpublished data).

Basic Tabulation for Mean[1] and Range[2]:			Sorted Tabulation for Mode[3]: Patients sorted in ascending order by No. of injections & Hash Totalling done next		
Patient ID	No. of injections	Range[1]	By patient index No. [now sorted by next column]	No. of injections received by each patient	Mode[2] (Hash Totalling Done)
1	2	3	1	2	4
1AA	*1*	Minimum	1AA	1	||
2BB	5		4DD	1	2
3CC	3		5EE	2	||
4DD	*1*	Minimum	6FF	2	2
5EE	2		3CC	3	|||
6FF	2		10KK	3	3
7GG	7		11LL	3	
8HH	*12*	Maximum	2BB	5	||
9JJ	8		14PP	5	4
					| 1
10KK	3		13NN	6	1
11LL	5		7GG	7	||
12MM	7		12MM	7	2
13NN	6		9JJ	8	1
14PP	5		8HH	12	12

[1]*Mean symbol* ($\bar{x}$), The central tendency as represented by the mean would be calculated differently:
The symbol of the mean is usually given by the symbol "($\bar{x}$)". The bar above the letter x, represents the mean of x number of values.
$\bar{x}$ = (Sum of values ÷ Number of values)
$\bar{x} = (x_1 + x_2 + x_3 + \ldots + x_n)/n$
[2]*Range* in the above series is 12 – 1 = 11 (12 being the maximum number of injections received and 1 being the minimum number of injections received.
[3]*Mode* is defined as the most common value in this tally table is found to be "3" and hence the *mode* is the value 3.
Median is identified by another manner of sorting, illustrated elsewhere.

■ MEAN DEVIATION OR AVERAGE DEVIATION

In statistics, *mean deviation* (also known as the mean absolute deviation) is a measure of dispersion that indicates the average distance between each data point and the mean of the data set. It provides insight into the variability or spread of the data [**Tables 7.3(a) and 7.3(b)**].

To calculate the mean deviation, follow these steps:
1. *Find the mean* of the data set.
2. *Calculate the absolute differences* between each data point and the mean.
3. *Compute the average* of these absolute differences.

Mathematically, it can be expressed as:

$$\text{Mean deviation} = \frac{1}{n}\sum_{i=1}^{n}|x_1 - \bar{x}|$$

where n is the number of data points, x_i represents each data point, and is the mean of the data set.

Illustration

The example in **Table 7.3** from a study of 2 types of cataract surgery, illustrates the calculation of the mean and standard deviation for Endothelial Cell Counts, Axial Lengths and intraocular pressure (IOP) measurements taken from various patients in FLACS Group and CPS Group. This example demonstrates how to calculate the mean and standard deviation, which are essential measures in descriptive statistics. The mean provides the average value of the data set, while the standard deviation indicates the spread or variability of the data around the mean.

■ VARIANCE

Variance is a statistical measure that quantifies the degree of spread or dispersion in a set of data points. It indicates how much the values in a data set differ from the mean (average) of the data set. A higher variance means that the data points are more spread out from the mean, while a lower variance indicates that they are closer to the mean.

$$\text{Variance} = \frac{1}{n-1}\sum_{i=1}^{n}(x_i - \bar{x})^2$$

Illustration

Among 10 patients presenting to the ophthalmic outpatient department (OPD), the intraocular pressure (IOP) noted was 15, 12, 14, 18, 21, 22, 25, 26, 14, 12.

Hence, the average of the above IOP is 17.9.
Calculating variance for the above data is 26.94.

TABLE 7.3(a): Standard deviation values in endothelial cell count, axial length, and IOP post cataract surgery (Effect of femtosecond laser-assisted cataract surgery for cataracts after pars plana vitrectomy: A prospective randomize).

	FLACS group (n = 47)	CPS group (n = 45)	p value
Age (year)	53.34 ± 8.44	52.80 ± 13.84	0.823
Sex:			0.848
Male	21	21	
Female	26	24	
Emery-Little nuclear cataract grade			0.981
Grade I	0	0	
Grade II	8	9	
Grade III	19	18	
Grade IV	16	14	
Grade V	4	4	
BCVA (logMAR)			0.428
<1	37	34	
<0.5	10	9	
<0.3	0	2	
The mean ECD (cells/mm^2)	2,561.87 ± 397.85	2,658.31 ± 311.89	0.200
AL (mm)	26.49 ± 2.61	27.28 ± 3.39	0.212
IOP (mm Hg)	15.54 ± 3.43	15.68 ± 3.34	0.841
Protopathy			0.046
RRD	36	33	
Diabetic retinopathy	3	7	
Macula hole	1	4	
Epiretinal membrane	7	1	

(AL: axial length; BCVA: best corrected visual acuity; CPS: conventional phacoemulsification; ECD: endothelial cell density; FLACS: femtosecond laser-assisted cataract surgery; IOP: intraocular pressure; logMAR: log of minimum angle of resolution; RRD: rhegmatogenous retinal detachment)

■ STANDARD DEVIATION

In statistics, the *standard deviation* is a measure of the amount of variation or dispersion of a set of values. It quantifies how much the values in a dataset deviate from the mean (average) of the dataset. A low standard deviation indicates that the values tend to be close to the mean, while a high standard deviation indicates that the values are spread out over a wider range **[Tables 7.3(a) and 7.3(b)]**.

$$\text{Standard deviation} = \sqrt{\frac{1}{n-1}\sum_{i=1}^{n}(x_i - \bar{x})^2}$$

TABLE 7.3(b): Explanation for **Table 7.3(a)** depicted.

Interpretation of the values of *standard deviation* in endothelial cell counts with respect to the femtosecond laser-assisted cataract surgery (FLACS) in the illustration	*Standard deviation* is a measure of the amount of variation or dispersion in a set of values. It quantifies how much the values in a dataset deviate from the mean (average) of the dataset. A low standard deviation indicates that the values tend to be close to the mean, while a high standard deviation indicates that the values are spread out over a wider range. In the context of endothelial cell counts with respect to FLACS, the standard deviation can provide insights into the variability of cell counts among patients who underwent the surgery. Here's how to interpret it: • *Low standard deviation*: If the standard deviation of endothelial cell counts is low, it means that the cell counts are relatively consistent across different patients. This suggests that the FLACS surgery has a predictable impact on endothelial cell counts, with most patients experiencing similar outcomes. • *High standard deviation*: If the standard deviation is high, it indicates that there is a wide range of endothelial cell counts among patients. This suggests that the impact of FLACS surgery on endothelial cell counts varies significantly from patient to patient, with some experiencing higher or lower counts than others

Illustration

The illustration is provided in **Tables 7.3(a) and 7.3(b)**.

■ VARIANCE VERSUS STANDARD DEVIATION

While both variance and standard deviation measure the spread of data, their interpretations and applications can differ slightly. Let us study two examples:
1. *Interpretation in the area of visual acuity measurements:*
    a. *Variance:*
        i. *Interpretation:* Variance gives you a sense of how much the data points differ from the mean, but it is in squared units, which can make it less intuitive.
        ii. *Example:* In our example, a variance of 0.0026 indicates the average squared deviation from the mean visual acuity **(Table 7.4)**.
    b. *Standard deviation:*
        i. *Interpretation:* Standard deviation is the square root of the variance, bringing the measure back to the original units of the data, making it more interpretable.

ii. *Example:* A standard deviation of 0.051 in visual acuity measurements tells us that, on average, the IOP values deviate from the mean by about 0.051 **(Table 7.4)**.
2. *Applicability:*
    a. *Variance:*
        i. *Use in statistical analysis:* Variance is often used in more complex statistical analyses, such as in the calculation of other statistical measures [e.g., analysis of variance (ANOVA)] and regression analysis).
        ii. *Example:* In ophthalmology research, variance might be used to compare the variability of visual acuity, IOP measurements between different groups of patients.
    b. *Standard deviation:*
        i. *Use in practical applications:* Standard deviation is more commonly used in practical applications because it is easier to interpret. It helps in understanding the consistency or variability of measurements.

TABLE 7.4: Interpretation in visual acuity measurements.

Visual acuity tests measure the clarity or sharpness of vision. Suppose we have visual acuity measurements (in logMAR units) from a group of patients • Patient 1: 0.1 • Patient 2: 0.2 • Patient 3: 0.15 • Patient 4: 0.05 • Patient 5: 0.1	*Calculate the mean (average) visual acuity:* • Mean = 0.12 logMAR • Variance = 0.0026 logMAR • Standard deviation = 0.051 logMAR *Interpretation and applicability* • *Variance:* In this example, the variance of 0.0026 logMAR indicates the average squared deviation from the mean visual acuity. This measure is useful in research settings to compare the variability of visual acuity across different patient groups or treatment conditions • *Standard deviation:* The standard deviation of 0.051 logMAR provides a more intuitive measure of the spread of visual acuity measurements around the mean. Clinicians can use this to understand the consistency of visual acuity results among patients, which is crucial for assessing the effectiveness of treatments or interventions By comparing the variance and standard deviation in visual acuity measurements, researchers and clinicians can gain insights into the variability and consistency of vision outcomes in different patient populations

ii. *Example:* Clinicians might use the standard deviation of IOP measurements to assess the consistency of a patient's IOP readings over time, which can be crucial for monitoring glaucoma progression.

Example Interpretation in Visual Acuity Measurements

Interpretation in visual acuity measurements is mentioned in **Table 7.4**.

■ SKEWNESS

Skewness is a measure of the asymmetry of the probability distribution of a real-valued random variable about its mean. It indicates whether the data points are skewed to the left (negative skewness) or the right (positive skewness) of the mean. Here are some key points about skewness **[Fig. 7.1 and Tables 7.5(a) and 7.5(b)]**:

- *Positive skewness:* The right tail is longer, and the mass of the distribution is concentrated on the left. This means that the mean is greater than the median.
- *Negative skewness:* The left tail is longer, and the mass of the distribution is concentrated on the right. This means that the mean is less than the median.
- *Zero skewness:* The tails on both sides of the mean balance out overall, indicating a symmetric distribution

For example, in a dataset of examination scores, if most students scored low but a few scored very high, the distribution would be positively skewed. Conversely, if most students scored high but a few scored very low, the distribution would be negatively skewed.

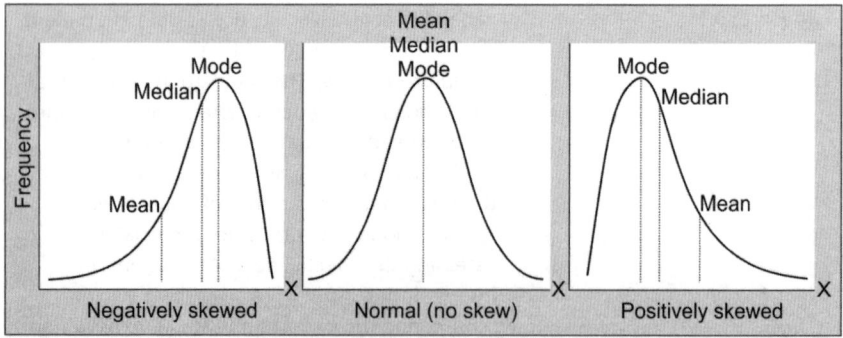

Fig. 7.1: In normally distributed data, mean = median = mode; in negatively skewed data, mean <median <mode—e.g., visual acuity outcomes following cataract surgery; in positively skewed data, mean > median > mode—e.g., intraocular pressure (IOP) distribution in population as age increases.

TABLE 7.5(a): Explanation for **Figure 7.1.**

In the context of intraocular pressure (IOP) readings, as age increases, the distribution of IOP values tends to become positively skewed	This can be due to several factors: • *Age-related changes:* As people age, there may be physiological changes in the eye that affect IOP. These changes can lead to a wider range of IOP values, with some individuals experiencing significantly higher IOP • *Increased variability:* Older populations may have more variability in their IOP readings due to a higher prevalence of eye conditions such as glaucoma, which can cause elevated IOP • *Outliers:* In older age groups, there may be more individuals with extremely high IOP values, which can pull the mean to the right, resulting in positive skewness In summary, positive skewness in IOP readings as age increases indicates that while most individuals have IOP values clustered around a lower range, there are a few individuals with significantly higher IOP values, leading to an asymmetric distribution

TABLE 7.5(b): Explanation for **Figure 7.1.**

An example of negative skewing can be observed in the distribution of visual acuity scores after a specific treatment	• We see that following cataract surgery, most patients achieve high visual acuity scores posttreatment, but a few patients have significantly lower scores, the distribution of these scores would be negatively skewed. This means that the majority of the data points (visual acuity scores) are clustered on the right side of the mean, with a long tail on the left side representing the few patients with lower scores • Negative skewness indicates that the mean is less than the median, and the mass of the distribution is concentrated on the right. This can be due to various factors, such as the effectiveness of the treatment for most patients, with only a few experiencing less favorable outcomes

■ KURTOSIS

Kurtosis is a statistical measure that describes the "tailedness" of a distribution. It indicates how often outliers occur in a dataset. Kurtosis is often measured in comparison to a normal distribution. Excess kurtosis is the kurtosis relative to a normal distribution, where a normal distribution has an excess kurtosis of 0.

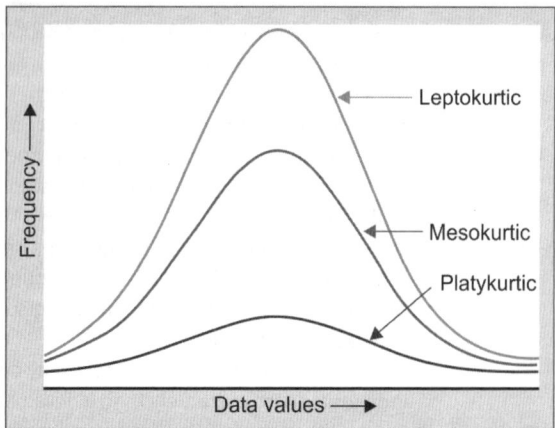

Fig. 7.2: Different types of Kurtosis.

There are three types of kurtosis:
1. *Mesokurtic:* This type of distribution has medium tails, meaning outliers are neither highly frequent nor highly infrequent. A normal distribution is an example of a mesokurtic distribution, with a kurtosis of approximately 3.
2. *Platykurtic:* This type of distribution has thin tails, meaning outliers are less frequent. Distributions with a kurtosis of <3 are considered platykurtic.
3. *Leptokurtic:* This type of distribution has fat tails, meaning outliers are more frequent. Distributions with a kurtosis of >3 are considered leptokurtic **(Fig. 7.2)**.

For example, in a dataset of examination scores, if the distribution is leptokurtic, it means there are more extreme scores (either very high or very low) compared to a normal distribution.

When dealing with data that has low, medium, or high kurtosis, different statistical tests can be applied to ensure accurate significance analysis **(Table 7.6)**. Here are some common tests:
- *Low kurtosis (platykurtic):*
  - *T-tests:* Suitable if the data is approximately normal
  - *ANOVA:* Used for comparing means across multiple groups if the data is normally distributed
- *Medium kurtosis (mesokurtic):*
  - *T-tests:* Appropriate for normally distributed data
  - *ANOVA:* Also suitable for normally distributed data
- *High kurtosis (leptokurtic):*
  - *Robust tests*: Such as the Welch's t-test, which is less sensitive to deviations from normality

TABLE 7.6: Illustrative tabulation of skew and kurtosis being tested for all variables prior to application of statistical significance tests.

Variable and its function	Delayed PPV (n = 12)			Same-day PPV (n = 23)			Skew/kurtosis[b] test		Shapiro-Wilk[b] test	
	Min	Md	Max	Min	Md	Max	adj χ^2	p value	Z	p value
Independent or confounding variables										
Age at final visit	58.13	81.99	97.03	62.79	85.65	99.45	8.63	0.013*	2.20	0.014*
VA logMAR OP pre-CS	0.176	0.438	1.602	0.176	0.477	2.204	10.88	0.004**	3.92	0.000***
VA Snellen OP pre-CS	20/800	20/55	20/30	20/3077	20/60	20/30	4.07	0.130	−1.64	0.950
VA logMAR non-OP pre-CS	0.000	0.176	0.544	0.000	0.301	1.000	12.44	0.002**	2.89	0.002**
VA Snellen non-OP pre-CS	20/70	20/30	20/20	20/200	20/40	20/20	0.95	0.623	−1.55	0.939
FU post-PPV (months)	5.93	53.28	113.37	3.07	36.57	123.50	2.83	0.243	1.86	0.031*
Total elapsed time (months)	6.33	56.57	115.30	3.07	36.57	123.50	2.85	0.240	1.89	0.030*
VA logMAR non-OP final	0.000	0.018	0.544	0.000	0.097	1.301	18.35	0.000***	4.19	0.000***
VA Snellen non-OP final	20/70	20/30	20/20	20/400	20/25	20/20	2.77	0.250	0.32	0.374
Dependent variables										
VA logMAR OP final	0.097	0.301	2.204	0.000	0.176	2.204	18.23	0.000***	5.05	0.000***
VA Snellen OP final	20/3200	20/40	20/25	20/3200	20/30	20/20	3.24	0.198	−0.39	0.651
Visual utility—better eye[a]	0.74	0.84	0.97	0.77	0.87	1.00	4.15	0.126	1.00	0.160
Visual utility—both eyes[a]	0.805	0.96	0.96	0.83	0.96	0.96	7.27	0.026*	3.04	0.001**
Diff MD glaucoma prog	−8.12	−6.37	−1.63	−3.35	−1.15	5.72	0.21	0.899	−0.63	0.737
Diff PSD glaucoma prog	0.11	0.895	6.11	−2.76	−0.85	0.31	10.38	0.006**	2.10	0.018*

Notes: *$P \leq 0.05$; **$P \leq 0.01$; ***$P \leq 0.001$; †$P \leq 0.15$.

[a]Visual utility analyses included 22 same-day patients. Visual utility—better eye: 1.00 = 20/20 bilaterally, permanently; 0.97 = 20/20 with 20/20 to 20/25 in the other eye, 0.92 = 20/20 with ≤20/40 in the other eye, 0.87 = 20/25, 0.84 = 20/30, 0.80 = 20/40, 0.77 = 20/50, 0.74 = 20/70.[16] Visual utility - both eyes: 0.96 = better eye 20/20 to 20/40 and worse eye >20/200, 0.88 = better eye 20/50 to 20/80 and worse eye >20/200, 0.83 = better eye 20/20 to 20/200, 0.88 = better eye 20/50 to 20/80 and worse eye <20/200;[17]
0.88 = better eye 20/50 to 20/80 and worse eye <20/200.[17]

[b]The null hypothesis for the skew/kurtosis test and the Shapiro-Wilk test is that the data come from a normal distribution.

(adj χ^2: adjusted chi-square statistic; Diff: differential; FU: follow-up time in months; Max: maximum; Md: median; Min: minimum; n: number of eyes; non-OP, nonoperated eye; OP: operated eye; post-PPV: after pars plana vitrectomy; PPV: pars plana vitrectomy; pre-CS: before cataract surgery; prog: progression; VA: visual acuity; Z: Z statistic)

- *Nonparametric tests*: Such as the Mann-Whitney U test or Kruskal-Wallis test, which do not assume normality and are less affected by outliers.

In general, when kurtosis is high, it indicates the presence of outliers, and robust or nonparametric tests are preferred to handle the deviations from normality.

It is sometimes possible to remove extreme data points (outliers) and then perform common statistical tests. However, this approach should be done with caution. Here are some considerations:

- *Identify outliers:* Use statistical methods to identify outliers, such as the IQR method or Z-scores.
- *Justify removal:* Ensure there is a valid reason for removing outliers. Outliers can sometimes provide important information about the data.
- *Impact on results:* Removing outliers can affect the results of your analysis. It is important to report both the results with and without outliers to provide a complete picture.
- *Alternative approaches:* Instead of removing outliers, consider using robust statistical methods that are less sensitive to outliers, such as the Mann-Whitney U test or robust regression techniques.

CONCLUSION

Considering the prevalence of outliers and deviations from normality in datasets, the choice of statistical methods becomes critical. Robust and nonparametric tests offer reliable alternatives to traditional parametric tests, ensuring the integrity of the analysis even in the presence of anomalies. While the removal of outliers can be considered, it must be approached with caution and justified appropriately. By leveraging these advanced statistical techniques, researchers can derive meaningful insights and maintain the validity of their findings.

BIBLIOGRAPHY

1. Helaly HA, Elkhawaga MH, El-mansy MS, Hassan MS. Studying the added effect of sum-of-segments biometry to modern intraocular lens power calculation formulas for short eyes. BMC Ophthalmology [Internet]. 2025 (cited 2025-02-12); 25(1). Available from: https://doi.org/10.1186/s12886-025-03896-1
2. Vanner EA, Stewart MW, Liesegang TJ, Bendel RE, Bolling JP, Hasan SA. A retrospective cohort study of clinical outcomes for intravitreal crystalline retained lens fragments after age-related cataract surgery: a comparison of same-day versus delayed vitrectomy. Clin Ophthalmol [Internet]. 2012 (cited 2012);6:1135-48. Available from: https://doi.org/10.2147/opth.S27564

CHAPTER 8

Probability and Distributions

Sunil Moreker, T Raveendra, Srinivasa Rao Pasala, Sowmya Peri

■ INTRODUCTION

As ophthalmologists, the intricate dance of numbers and the probabilities they represent play a crucial role in our practice. Whether we are evaluating the likelihood of a patient developing an ocular condition or predicting the success rate of a surgical procedure, a deep understanding of probability and distribution is indispensable. By harnessing statistical tools, we can make informed decisions that enhance patient care and optimize treatment outcomes, ensuring that our interventions are both precise and effective.

One key application of probability in ophthalmology is in the assessment of disease prevalence and incidence. For instance, understanding the probability of developing conditions such as glaucoma or macular degeneration based on hereditary factors or demographic data allows us to implement proactive screening and early intervention strategies. This not only improves patient prognosis but also optimizes resource allocation within our practices.

Moreover, probability plays a vital role in evaluating the risks and benefits of various treatment options. By analyzing clinical trial data and patient outcomes, we can estimate the likelihood of success and potential complications for different surgical techniques or therapeutic interventions. This empowers us to tailor our recommendations to each patient's unique circumstances, thus enhancing the overall quality of care.

In addition, statistical distributions assist us in interpreting diagnostic test results. Understanding the distribution of test values in healthy versus diseased populations helps us to determine the sensitivity and specificity of these tests. This, in turn, guides our diagnostic accuracy and ensures that we provide timely and appropriate management for our patients.

Ultimately, the mastery of probability and distribution equips us with the analytical skills necessary to navigate the complexities of modern ophthalmology. By leveraging these concepts, we can continuously improve our clinical practices, contribute to the advancement of our field, and ultimately improve the vision and lives of our patients.

■ PROBABILITY

Probability is a measure of the likelihood that a particular event will occur. It quantifies the uncertainty associated with random events and is expressed as a number between 0 and 1, where 0 indicates that the event will not occur and 1 indicates that the event will certainly occur. The formula for probability is given by:

$$P(E) = \frac{\text{Number of favorable outcomes}}{\text{Total number of outcomes}}$$

For example, when flipping a coin, the probability of getting heads is 0.5, as there is one favorable outcome (heads) out of two possible outcomes (heads or tails).

Probability is a fundamental concept in statistics and is used to make inferences about populations based on sample data. It helps in predicting the likelihood of various outcomes and is widely applied in fields such as finance, insurance, medicine, and engineering **(Table 8.1)**.

Examples like prevalence = Probability of having a disease from hereditary/other factors, etc.

Illustration-1

Ophthalmologists use probability to predict the success rates of various procedures. For example, the probability of achieving 20/20 vision after laser-assisted in situ keratomileusis (LASIK) surgery is based on preoperative measurements and patient characteristics.

Probability helps in estimating the likelihood of certain eye diseases within a population. For instance, determining the probability of developing glaucoma based on age, family history, and other risk factors.

TABLE 8.1: Representing probability with Maretz et al.

Infectious keratitis in Western New York: A 10-year review of patient demographics, clinical management, and treatment failure

Importance of probability	• Probability is essential for making informed decisions in uncertain situations, predicting outcomes, mitigating risks, and optimizing results. In medicine, it helps determine disease likelihood, treatment success, and complications. In finance, it predicts market trends and assesses investment risks. Engineers use probability for quality control, reliability analysis, and risk assessment • Overall, probability's importance lies in its ability to analyze data, make predictions, and guide decisions effectively (p-value) • *In this article, probability is like*: We sought to understand if certain patient characteristics were associated with a higher probability of presenting with a probably sight-threatening (PST) ulcer

Applications of Probability in Ophthalmology

Probability plays a crucial role in various aspects of ophthalmology, enhancing decision-making, diagnostics, and treatment outcomes. Here are some key applications:

- *Diagnosis of eye conditions:* Probability is used to assess the likelihood of various eye conditions, such as glaucoma, macular degeneration, and cataracts, based on risk factors, such as age, genetics, lifestyle, and clinical measurements. This helps ophthalmologists in early detection and timely intervention.
- *Treatment success rates:* By analyzing historical data and patient characteristics, ophthalmologists can predict the probability of success for different treatments. For instance, the likelihood of achieving 20/20 vision after LASIK surgery can be estimated, allowing patients to make informed decisions.
- *Clinical trials:* Probability is fundamental in designing and analyzing clinical trials for new medications and surgical techniques. It helps in determining sample sizes, evaluating outcomes, and establishing the efficacy and safety of new interventions.
- *Predictive modeling:* Probabilistic models are used to predict disease progression and response to treatment. For example, predicting the progression of diabetic retinopathy based on blood sugar levels and other health parameters enables personalized treatment plans.
- *Risk assessment:* Probability aids in assessing the risk of complications during and after eye surgeries. By understanding the probability of adverse events, ophthalmologists can take preventive measures and manage patient expectations effectively.
- *Public health planning:* Epidemiological studies use probability to estimate the prevalence and incidence of eye diseases in different populations. This information is crucial for public health planning, resource allocation, and implementing preventive measures.
- *Personalized medicine:* Probability is used to tailor treatments based on individual patient profiles. For instance, the probability of success for specific intraocular lenses in cataract surgery can be determined based on the patient's eye measurements and lifestyle needs.

■ PROBABILITY DISTRIBUTIONS

In statistics, distribution refers to the way in which the values of a dataset are spread or dispersed. It describes the frequency or probability of each value or range of values occurring in the dataset. Understanding the distribution of data is crucial for interpreting and analyzing statistical results, as it provides insights into patterns, trends, and anomalies within the data **(Flowchart 8.1)**.

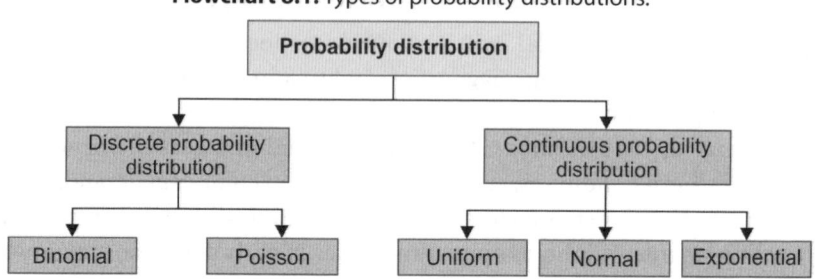

Flowchart 8.1: Types of probability distributions.

The distribution of data is often visualized using graphs such as histograms, probability density functions (PDFs), or cumulative distribution functions, which help to clearly illustrate the shape and spread of the data. Understanding the distribution is essential for selecting appropriate statistical tests, estimating probabilities, and making data-driven decisions.

The characteristics of the variable, as outlined in **Chapter 7**, along with the distribution of the data within the dataset, must be examined and classified. This is essential for selecting the appropriate statistical test for accurate interpretation of the data and results.

In the realm of probability and statistics, distributions play a pivotal role in understanding and interpreting data. They describe how values in a dataset are spread, providing critical insights into patterns, trends, and potential anomalies. Different types of distributions are used based on the nature of the data and the specific analysis required.

Various types of distributions are utilized to model different kinds of data, which are discussed further.

Discrete Probability Distributions

Discrete probability distributions are used for variables that can take on a finite or countably infinite number of distinct values.

Binomial Distribution

This distribution represents the number of successes in a fixed number of independent binary (success/failure) experiments. It is particularly useful in scenarios where outcomes can be categorized into two distinct groups. For instance, the success rate of a surgical procedure like cataract surgery can be categorized as an outcome better than 6/18 in Yes or No **(Table 8.2)**. Alternatively, the rate of endophthalmitis can be modeled as a negative binomial distribution.

TABLE 8.2: Probability of getting a successful visual outcome 6/18.

Procedure	Success rate	Outcome
Cataract surgery	Better than 6/18	Yes or no

Poisson Distribution

The Poisson distribution models the number of events occurring within a fixed interval of time or space, given a constant mean rate and independence of events. This distribution is commonly used to predict the occurrence of rare events, such as the number of complication cases during a particular period in an ophthalmology clinic.

Continuous Probability Distributions

Unlike discrete distributions, continuous probability distributions describe variables that can take on an infinite number of values within a given range. These distributions are essential for modeling and analyzing continuous data.

Uniform Distribution

The uniform distribution is a type of continuous probability distribution where all intervals of the same length are equally probable. It is often used when each outcome in a range is equally likely, such as the time of arrival of patients within a given hour in a clinic.

Eye color distribution in a diverse population is also a uniformly distributed factor, assuming that each eye color has an equal likelihood of appearing within the population. This makes uniform distribution a versatile tool for various real-world applications.

Exponential Distribution

The exponential distribution models the time between events in a Poisson process, where events occur continuously and independently at a constant average rate. This distribution is particularly useful in predicting the time until the next occurrence of an event, such as the time between patient arrivals in an emergency room.

The exponential distribution is used in survival analysis to model the time until an event, such as cure or relapse, occurs. This is particularly useful in clinical trials and epidemiological studies, where understanding the timing of such events can inform treatment decisions and policymaking. For example, in the context of eye health, the exponential distribution could help predict the time between follow-up visits for patients undergoing treatment for chronic eye conditions.

Normal Distribution

The normal distribution, also known as the Gaussian distribution, is one of the most widely used continuous probability distributions. It describes data that clusters around a mean or average value, creating a bell-shaped curve.

This distribution is crucial in various statistical analyses, such as determining the distribution of heights, blood pressure readings, and test scores in a population.

A *normal distribution*, also known as a Gaussian distribution, is a continuous probability distribution that is symmetrical and bell-shaped, describing how the values of a variable are distributed. In a normal distribution, most of the data points cluster around the mean (average), and the probabilities for values further away from the mean taper off equally in both directions.

Mathematically, the PDF of a normal distribution is given by:

$$f(x) = \frac{1}{\sqrt{2\pi}\sigma} e^{-\frac{1}{2}\left(\frac{x-\mu}{\sigma}\right)^2}$$

Importance of Normal Distribution

The normal distribution is important in many fields, including ophthalmology and broader medical research, due to its unique properties and applications. One key aspect of the normal distribution is its utility in statistical inference. Many statistical tests, such as the t-test and analysis of variance (ANOVA), are based on the assumption of normality, which allows researchers to make reliable inferences about a population from sample data.

In clinical trials, the normal distribution helps in understanding the variability in patient responses to treatments. It enables researchers to model the distribution of treatment effects and distinguish between true treatment effects and random variation. This is crucial for determining the efficacy and safety of new medical interventions.

Moreover, normal distribution is foundational in the development of predictive models. Because many biological processes exhibit normal distribution patterns, these models can accurately predict disease progression and treatment responses, leading to better patient care and personalized medicine.

In risk assessment, normal distribution aids ophthalmologists in estimating the likelihood of various outcomes, thus enhancing decision-making and patient management. For example, understanding the distribution of intraocular pressure (IOP) in a population can help identify patients at risk of glaucoma.

Overall, normal distribution is a cornerstone of statistical analysis and decision-making in ophthalmology and other medical fields, providing a robust framework for understanding and managing variability in clinical and public health contexts.

Characteristics of Normal Distribution

The normal distribution, also referred to as the Gaussian distribution, possesses several distinct characteristics that make it a fundamental concept in statistics and probability.

- *Symmetry:* The normal distribution is perfectly symmetrical about its mean. This implies that the left half of the distribution is a mirror image of the right half.
- *Bell-shaped curve*: The shape of the normal distribution is bell-shaped, with the highest point at the mean, gradually tapering off as you move away from the mean in both directions **(Fig. 8.1)**.
- *Mean, median, and mode*: In a normal distribution, the mean, median, and mode are all equal and located at the center of the distribution.
- *Asymptotic nature*: The tails of the distribution curve approach the horizontal axis but never touch it, extending infinitely in both directions.
- *Empirical rule*: Also known as the 68-95-99.7 rule, this states that approximately 68% of the data falls within one standard deviation of the mean, 95% within two standard deviations, and 99.7% within three standard deviations.
- *Unimodal*: The normal distribution has a single peak, meaning it is unimodal. This peak occurs at the mean of distribution.
- *Defined by mean and standard deviation*: The shape of a normal distribution is determined entirely by its mean (μ) and standard deviation (σ). The mean indicates the center of the distribution, while the standard deviation measures the spread or dispersion of the data.

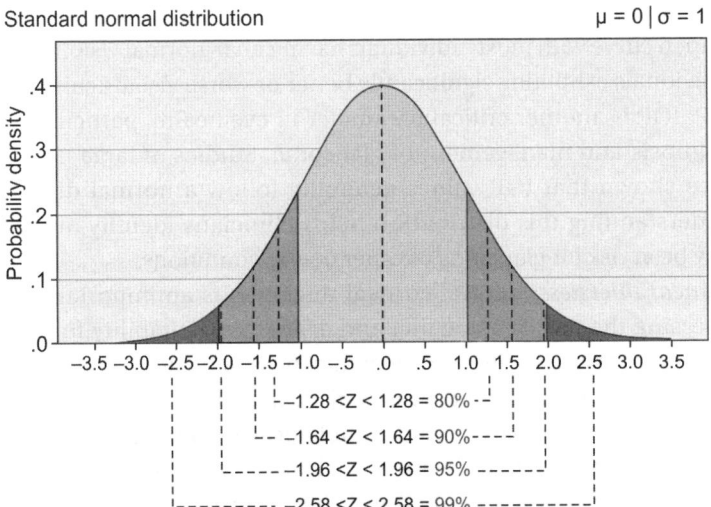

Fig. 8.1: Normal curve or Gaussian curve.

These characteristics make the normal distribution a powerful tool for statistical analysis and interpretation, facilitating the understanding and prediction of various phenomena across numerous fields.

Skewed Distribution

When data points are not symmetrically distributed around the mean, they exhibit skewness. Skewness can be either negative (left-skewed) or positive (right-skewed).

- Negative skewness, or left-skewness—means that the tail on the left side of the distribution is longer or fatter than the right side. This often indicates that there are more extreme low values in the dataset. For example, income distributions in many populations tend to be left-skewed, as a majority may have similar income levels, but there are fewer instances of extremely low incomes.
- Positive skewness, or right-skewness—implies that the tail on the right side of the distribution is longer or fatter than the left side. This suggests more extremely high values in the dataset. An example of this could be the distribution of exam scores, where a majority score moderately well, but a few individuals achieve exceptionally high scores.

Understanding skewness helps in identifying the direction and relative magnitude of data deviations from a normal distribution, which can be crucial for statistical analysis and decision-making.

Illustrations:

- *Visual acuity measurement:* Visual acuity, a fundamental measurement in ophthalmology, often follows a normal distribution in the general population. When testing large groups, the results typically form a bell-shaped curve with most individuals having near-normal vision, and fewer individuals exhibiting significantly better or worse visual acuity.
- *IOP:* IOP is another critical parameter in eye health, particularly in the diagnosis and management of glaucoma. Studies of large populations have shown that IOP values generally follow a normal distribution. Understanding this distribution helps clinicians identify outliers who may be at risk for glaucoma or other ocular conditions.
- *Corneal thickness:* Central corneal thickness is an important factor in assessing the risk of glaucoma and evaluating suitability for refractive surgery. Measurements of corneal thickness in healthy populations tend to be normally distributed. This statistical insight aids in distinguishing between normal variations and pathological conditions.
- *Refractive errors:* Refractive errors such as myopia (nearsightedness) and hyperopia (farsightedness) often exhibit normal distribution patterns within populations. Recognizing these patterns helps in understanding

the prevalence and distribution of these conditions, enabling better public health strategies and resource allocation.
- *Retinal nerve fiber layer thickness:* The thickness of the retinal nerve fiber layer is assessed using optical coherence tomography (OCT) and is essential in diagnosing and monitoring glaucoma. Normal population studies show that these thickness measurements usually form a normal distribution curve. This distribution helps in setting reference ranges that are critical for clinical decisions.
- *Lens thickness:* The thickness of the crystalline lens changes with age and can affect refractive status and risk of cataracts. Studies have shown that lens thickness measurements in various age groups form a normal distribution. This statistical pattern assists in age-related eye condition research and treatment planning.

CONCLUSION

In summary, the assessment of IOP, corneal thickness, refractive errors, retinal nerve fiber layer thickness, and lens thickness all exhibit normal distribution patterns within populations. These insights into the statistical distributions are invaluable for clinicians to differentiate between normal anatomical variations and pathological conditions. They play a crucial role in the prevention, diagnosis, and management of various ocular diseases, ultimately contributing to improved patient outcomes and advancing the field of ophthalmology.

BIBLIOGRAPHY

1. Maretz C, Atlas J, Shah S, Sohn MB, Wozniak RAF. Frontiers | Infectious keratitis in Western New York: a 10-year review of patient demographics, clinical management, and treatment failure. Front Ophthalmol [Internet]. 2024 (cited 2024/12/11);4. Available from: https://doi.org/10.3389/fopht.2024.1469966

CHAPTER 9

Correlation and Regression

Krishna Prasad Pallem, Srinivasa Rao Pasala

■ INTRODUCTION

As ophthalmologists, we often encounter patients with a multitude of visual and systemic conditions that seem interrelated. The study of correlation and regression analysis enables us to understand and interpret these relationships more precisely. By recognizing patterns and associations between different variables, such as intraocular pressure (IOP) and the progression of glaucoma, or the correlation between blood sugar levels and diabetic retinopathy, we can make informed decisions that enhance patient care.

Regression analysis plays a crucial role in intraocular lens (IOL) power calculations. By applying these statistical methods, we can accurately predict the optimal IOL power for individual patients based on variables such as axial length, corneal curvature, and anterior chamber depth. This ensures that patients receive the best possible visual outcomes following cataract surgery.

Moreover, multiple regression analysis is invaluable in other ophthalmic situations. For instance, when investigating the factors influencing the progression of age-related macular degeneration, we can analyze the impact of various predictors such as genetic markers, lifestyle factors, and environmental influences. This comprehensive approach allows us to develop more effective strategies for preventing and managing ocular diseases.

Understanding the nuances of correlation and regression equips us with the ability to critically analyze medical literature, ensuring that we apply evidence-based practices in our daily work. By leveraging these statistical methods, we contribute to the advancement of ophthalmic science and, ultimately, to the betterment of our patients' ocular health.

■ CORRELATION ANALYSIS

Correlation is a statistical measure that describes the degree to which two variables move in relation to each other. It quantifies the strength and direction of a linear relationship between two variables, expressed by the correlation coefficient, which ranges from –1 to 1.

Types of Correlations

- *Positive correlation:* When two variables move in the same direction, i.e., as one variable increases, the other variable also increases, and vice versa. For instance, the correlation between the amount of time spent studying and exam scores is often positive **(Fig. 9.1A)**.

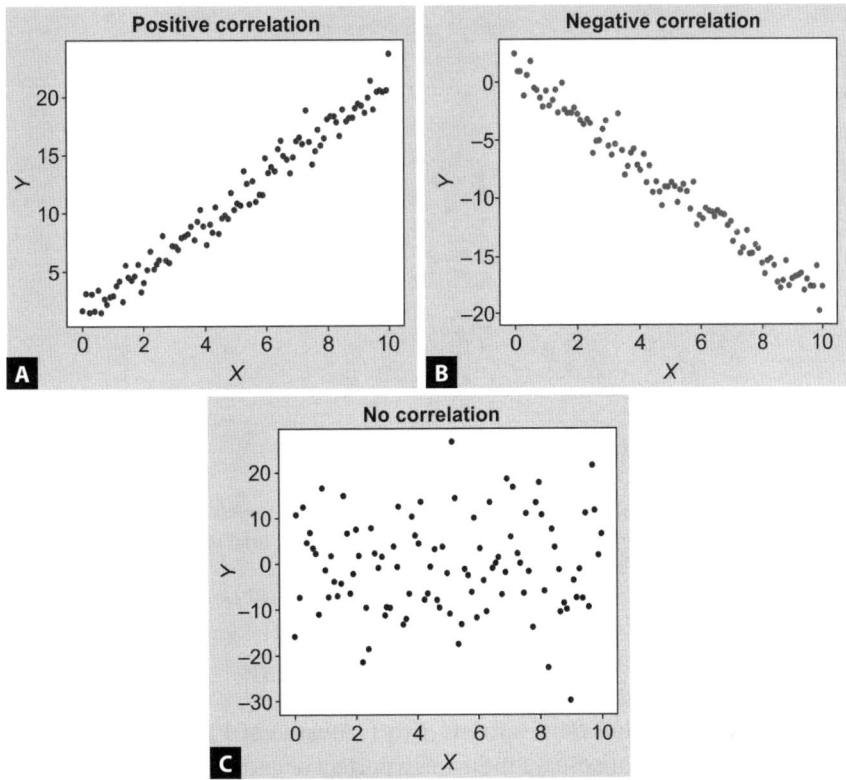

Figs. 9.1A to C: Correlation representation.

- *Negative correlation:* When two variables move in opposite directions, i.e., as one variable increases, the other variable decreases. An example of this is the correlation between the number of hours spent watching TV and academic performance **(Fig. 9.1B)**.
- *Zero correlation:* When there is no relationship between the two variables, meaning the movement of one variable does not predict the movement of the other. For instance, there might be zero correlation between the number of books read and the amount of rainfall in a year **(Fig. 9.1C)**.

Understanding the type of correlation is crucial for interpreting the data accurately and making informed decisions based on statistical analysis.

METHODS OF MEASURING OF CORRELATION COEFFICIENT

Karl–Pearson Correlation Coefficient

Karl–Pearson correlation coefficient: This is the most widely used method for measuring the degree of relationship between two variables **(Fig. 9.2)**. It is also known as the Pearson product-moment correlation coefficient.

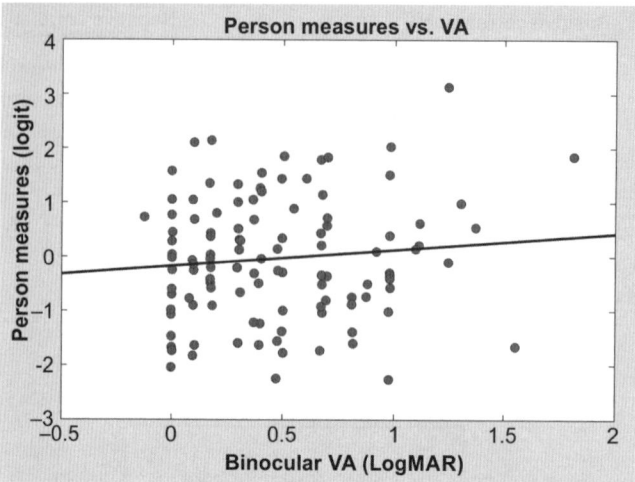

Fig. 9.2: Person measures (gray circles) plotted against logMAR binocular visual acuity (VA). The equation for the linear regression line (black line) is y = 0.3x − 0.18.

$$r = \frac{n(\Sigma xy) - (\Sigma x)(\Sigma y)}{\sqrt{[n\Sigma x_2 - (\Sigma x)^2][n\Sigma y^2 - (\Sigma y)^2]}}$$

The resulting value ranges from −1 to 1. A value of 1 indicates a perfect positive linear relationship, −1 indicates a perfect negative linear relationship, and 0 indicates no linear relationship. The Pearson correlation coefficient assumes that the relationship between the variables is linear and that the variables are normally distributed.

Illustration

Figure 9.2 depicts the Karl Pearson correlation coefficient between the binocular visual acuity (VA) and person Measures (M. et al., 2024/06/01).

Spearman Correlation Coefficient

The Spearman correlation coefficient comes into play while assessing the correlation between two ranked, i.e., qualitative ordinal data.

The *Spearman correlation coefficient*, also known as Spearman's rho (ρ), is a nonparametric measure of rank correlation. It assesses the strength and direction of the association between two ranked variables. Unlike Pearson's correlation, which measures linear relationships, Spearman's correlation evaluates monotonic relationships, whether linear or not **(Fig. 9.3)**.

$$r_s = 1 - \frac{6\Sigma d^2}{n(n^2 - 1)}$$

Here is a brief overview:
- *Calculation:* Spearman's correlation is calculated by converting the raw scores of the variables into ranks and then computing the Pearson correlation coefficient between these ranks.
- *Range:* The coefficient ranges from −1 to 1. A value of +1 indicates a perfect positive monotonic relationship, −1 indicates a perfect negative monotonic relationship, and 0 indicates no monotonic relationship.
- *Sensitivity:* Spearman's correlation is less sensitive to outliers compared to Pearson's correlation because it uses ranks instead of raw data values.

Fig. 9.3 illustrates the Spearman correlation concept with values of IOP's and Visual acuities being measured. The VA values represented as fractions (e.g., 20/40, 20/20), and the IOP values are constant at 18 mm Hg. The Spearman correlation coefficient is not defined in this case because of the intraocular pressure is shown as constant for all values of Visual acuity.

All values of that variable will have the same rank.

This results in zero variance for that variable.

Since correlation involves dividing by the product of the standard deviations (or rank variances), the denominator becomes zero, making the correlation undefined.

- *VA and contrast sensitivity:* Researchers often investigate the relationship between VA and contrast sensitivity in patients with various eye

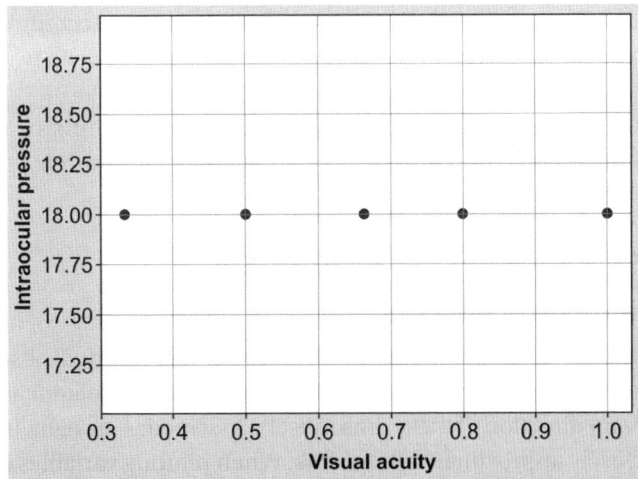

Fig. 9.3: In this example, the visual acuity values are represented as fractions (e.g., 20/40, 20/20), and the intraocular pressure values are constant at 18 mm Hg. The Spearman correlation coefficient is not defined in this case because the intraocular pressure is constant and unchanging.

conditions. For instance, a study might rank patients based on their VA and contrast sensitivity scores, then use the Spearman correlation coefficient to determine if there is a significant association between these two variables.
- *Dry eye symptoms and tear film stability*: Another example is examining the correlation between the severity of dry eye symptoms and the stability of the tear film. Patients could be ranked based on their symptom severity and tear film breakup time, and the Spearman correlation coefficient would help assess the strength and direction of the relationship between these ranks.

■ REGRESSION ANALYSIS

We have studied correlation analysis, which measures the direction and the strength of the relationship between two or more variables. However, in regression analysis, we can estimate or predict the value of one variable from the given value of the other variable. The relationship between IOP and age is examined to determine if age influences the risk of glaucoma.

Regression analysis helps us to estimate one variable, or the independent variable. In other words, we can estimate the value of one variable, provided that the value of the other variable is given. For Instance, in studying the changes in age leads how to change the IOP. The statistical method that helps us to estimate the unknown value of one variable from the known value of the related variable is called *regression*.

In Biostatistics, "regression technique" is applicable where two or more relative variables have a tendency to go back to the mean. According to Blair, "Regression is the measure of the average relationship between two or more variables in terms of the original units of the data."

Ya-Lun-Chow stated that "regression analysis attempts to establish the nature of the relationship between variables and thereby provide a mechanism for prediction or forecasting."

■ TYPES OF REGRESSION ANALYSIS

Linear Regression Analysis

To determine the relationship between two variables, individual observations are depicted as dots in a scatter diagram. If a significant correlation is present, the nature and direction of these dots must be assessed. A straight line is then drawn to closely approximate all the dots. When plotting variables (X and Y) on a scatter diagram, two "lines of best fit" can be created, passing through the plotted points. These lines are referred to as regression lines, and the equations derived from them are called regression equations **(Fig. 9.4 and Table 9.1)**.

The statistical analysis employed to find out the exact position of the straight line or lines is known as the "linear regression."

Polynomial Regression

Polynomial regression is an extension of linear regression, used when the relationship between the independent variable (X) and the dependent variable (Y) is not linear. Instead of fitting a straight line, polynomial

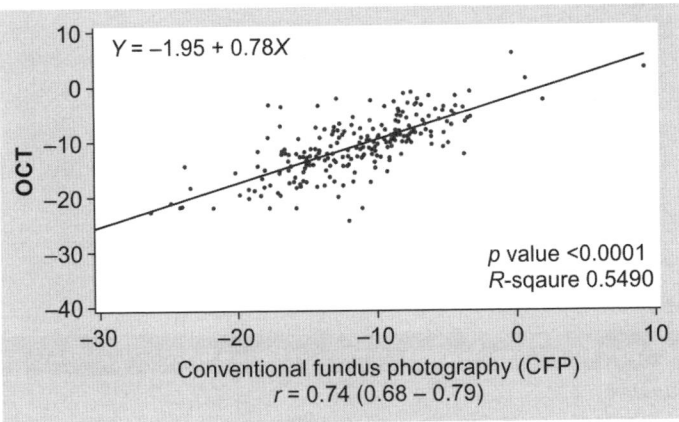

Fig. 9.4: Linear regression.

TABLE 9.1: Explaining the above linear regression **Figure 9.4**.	
In a study researcher mentioned about linear regression is titled "measurements of objective cyclotorsion in a population of healthy children"	
Linear regression	In multivariate linear regression with covariates, only AXL was an important predictor of DFA measured with CFP
(AXL: average axial length; CFP: conventional fundus photography; DFA: disc-center-fovea angle)	

regression fits a curved line to the data points. This method is particularly useful when data shows a curvilinear trend. Polynomial regression equations can include quadratic (squared) or higher-order terms of the independent variable, allowing for more complex relationships to be modeled.

In polynomial regression, the degree of the polynomial indicates the highest power of the independent variable in the equation. For example, a second-degree polynomial regression (quadratic regression) would include terms such as X and X^2, while a third-degree polynomial regression (cubic regression) would include terms such as X, X^2, and X^3. By incorporating

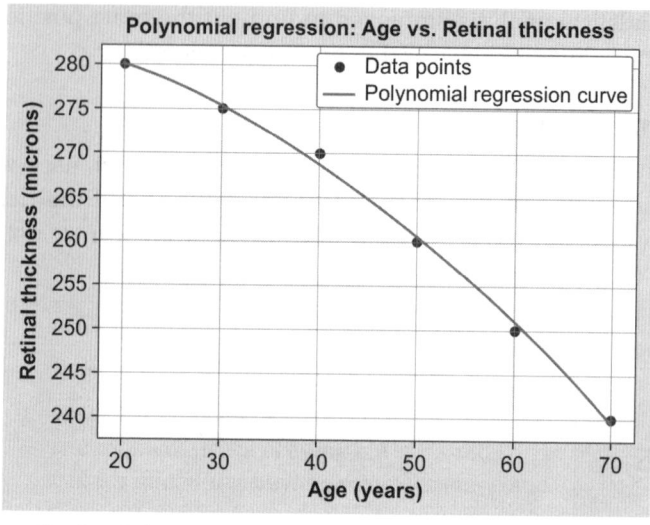

Fig. 9.5: Polynomial regression for age and retinal thickness.

BOX 9.1: Explanation for polynomial regression **Figure 9.5**.

In this diagram:
- The black dots represent the sample data points
- The gray curve represents the fitted polynomial regression model, showing how retinal thickness decreases with age in a nonlinear manner

Polynomial regression helps capture complex relationships between variables, making it useful in ophthalmology for modeling age-related changes in ocular measurements

---

these higher-degree terms, polynomial regression captures the nonlinear relationship between the variables more accurately **(Fig. 9.5 and Box 9.1)**.

Applications of polynomial regression are vast and can be seen in various fields such as economics, biology, and engineering. For instance, it can be used to model the growth rate of a species over time, where the relationship between time and population size is not simply linear but more complex. Additionally, polynomial regression can be used in finance to analyze the relationship between time and stock prices, which often exhibit cyclical patterns.

Logistic Regression

Logistic regression is a statistical method used when the dependent variable is categorical, often binary. Unlike linear regression, which predicts a continuous outcome, logistic regression predicts the probability of an event occurring by fitting data to a logistic curve. This method is particularly useful when the outcome is dichotomous, such as yes/no, success/failure, or presence/absence.

The logistic regression model estimates the probability that a given input point belongs to a specific category. The relationship between the independent variables (predictors) and the dependent variable (outcome) is modeled using the logistic function, also known as the sigmoid function. This function converts any real-valued number into a value between 0 and 1, representing the probability of the outcome **(Fig. 9.6 and Table 9.2)**.

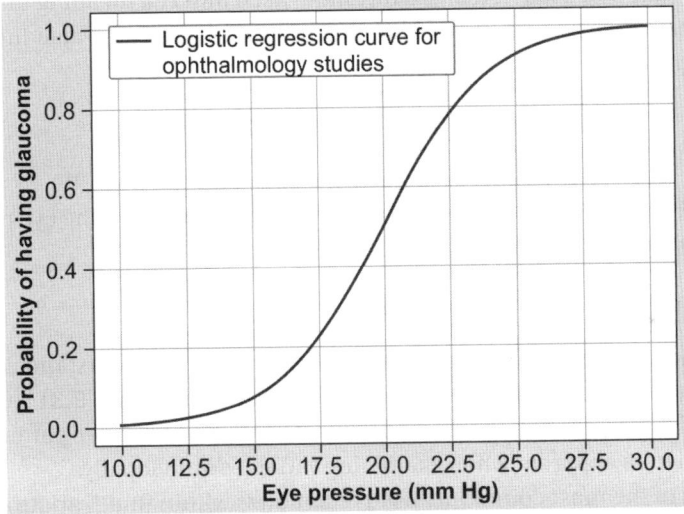

Fig. 9.6: Logistic regression curve presenting the relation between eye pressure and probability of having glaucoma.

TABLE 9.2: Explaining about logistic regression of **Figure 9.6**.	
In a study having the association of race with thyroid eye disease presentation and outcomes.	
Explaining about multiple logistic regression	Moreover, multiple logistic regression can identify interaction effects between predictors, revealing complex relationships that might be overlooked in simpler analyses. This capability is particularly beneficial in medical research, where the interplay between genetic, environmental, and lifestyle factors often shapes health outcomes. Thus, in the context of thyroid eye disease, multiple logistic regression not only elucidates the role of race but also aids in understanding how various factors collectively influence disease dynamics

Mathematically, the logistic regression model is represented as:

$$P(Y=1|X) = \frac{1}{[1+e-(\beta_0+\beta_1 x_1+\beta_2 x_2+...+\beta_n x_n]}$$

where $P(Y = 1|X)$ is the probability that the dependent variable Y equals 1 given the predictors $X_1, X_2, ..., X_n$; β_0 is the intercept term; $\beta_1, \beta_2, ..., \beta_n$ are the coefficients of the predictors; and e is the base of the natural logarithm.

Illustration (Fig. 9.6)

In this example, we assume that the x-axis represents eye pressure (measured in mm Hg), and the y-axis represents the probability of having glaucoma. The logistic function used here has a threshold at 20 mm Hg, meaning that as the eye pressure increases, the probability of having glaucoma also increases. The logistic function is defined as:

$$P(Y=1|x) = \frac{1}{1+e-(x-20)/2}$$

where $P(Y = 1|x)$ is the probability of having glaucoma given the eye pressure x, and e is the base of the natural logarithm.

■ MULTIVARIATE ANALYSIS

Multivariate analysis is a statistical technique used to understand relationships between multiple variables simultaneously **(Table 9.3)**. It allows researchers to analyze more complex data sets and uncover patterns that would not be apparent when examining variables individually.

One of the most commonly used techniques within multivariate analysis is multiple regression. Multiple regression is a statistical method that models the relationship between *a dependent variable and two or more independent variables.* By considering multiple predictors simultaneously, it provides a more comprehensive understanding of the factors influencing the outcome.

TABLE 9.3: Categories of multivariate analysis.

Category	Application
Disease progression and risk factors	Analyzing factors affecting disease progression, treatment efficacy, genetic expression, or quality of life, and identifying which are likely associated or not associated
Treatment efficacy	Evaluating the outcomes of medical treatments by considering multiple influencing factors
Genetic studies	Studying the relationship between genetic mutations and clinical manifestations

This approach not only helps in determining the strength and nature of the relationships but also allows for the control of confounding variables, leading to more accurate and reliable results.

We are not including complex multivariate analyses involving multiple dependent and independent variables, as these are beyond the scope of this work.

Applications in Ophthalmology

- *Disease progression and risk factors*:
  - *Glaucoma*: Multivariate analysis helps identify risk factors for glaucoma progression by analyzing variables such as intraocular pressure, age, and corneal thickness.
  - *Diabetic retinopathy:* It is used to study the impact of various factors such as blood sugar levels, duration of diabetes, and blood pressure on the progression of diabetic retinopathy.
- *Treatment efficacy:*
  - *Cataract surgery:* Multivariate techniques evaluate the outcomes of cataract surgery by considering factors, such as surgical technique, patient age, and preexisting conditions.
  - *Macular degeneration:* Analyzing the effectiveness of different treatments for macular degeneration by considering variables such as treatment type, patient demographics, and genetic factors
- *Genetic studies:*
  - *Retinitis pigmentosa:* Multivariate analysis is used to study the relationship between genetic mutations and clinical manifestations of retinitis pigmentosa, helping to identify potential genetic markers for the disease.
- *Visual function and quality of life:*
  - *VA:* It helps in understanding how various factors such as age, refractive errors, and ocular diseases affect VA and overall quality of life.
  - *Patient-reported outcomes:* Multivariate analysis is used to analyze patient-reported outcomes and satisfaction with treatments, providing a comprehensive view of treatment impact.

Multiple Regression

Multiple regression is a statistical technique used to understand the relationship between one dependent variable and two or more independent variables. It helps in predicting the value of the dependent variable based on the values of the independent variables **(Fig. 9.7 and Table 9.4)**.

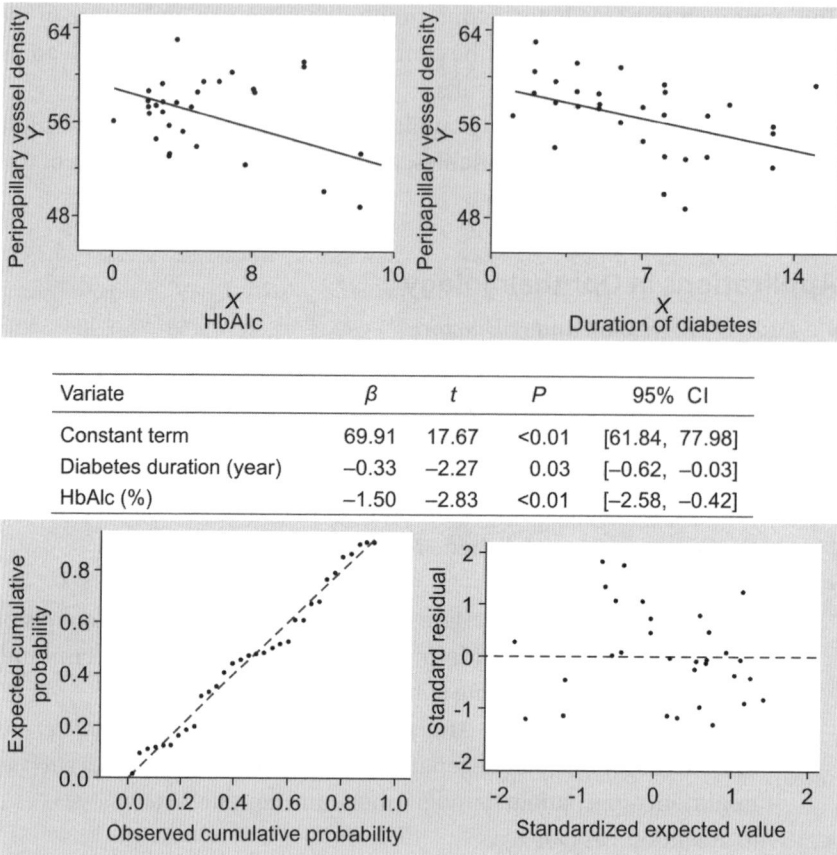

Fig. 9.7: Scatter plots representing negative linear relationship of glycated hemoglobin (HbA1c) and duration of diabetes (independent variables) with peripapillary vessel density (dependent variable) (Li & Wang, 2020/01/01).

TABLE 9.4: Explaining the above **Figure 9.7**.

Significance of multiple regression in the above example	<ul><li>Multiple regression analysis of peripapillary vessel density and systemic factors. Scatter plots of peripapillary vessel density and systemic factors show that the duration of diabetes and glycated hemoglobin (HbA1c) have a negative linear relationship with peripapillary vessel density</li><li>Other systemic factors, such as triglycerides, cholesterol, high-density lipoprotein, and low-density lipoprotein, do not exhibit a clear linear relationship with peripapillary density and were therefore excluded from the linear regression analyses. However, if one were to hypothesize potential *p*-values for these factors, it would be reasonable to expect nonsignificant values ($p > 0.05$), indicating that there is no statistically significant association between these systemic factors and peripapillary density in this particular dataset or study context</li></ul>

Key Concepts

- *Dependent variable (Y):* The outcome or the variable you are trying to predict or explain.
- *Independent Variables $(X_1, X_2, ... X_n)$:* The predictors or factors that you believe have an impact on the dependent variable.

Multiple Regression Equation

The general form of the multiple regression equation is:

$$Y = \beta_0 + \beta_1 X_1 + \beta_2 X_2 + ... + \beta n X_n + \varepsilon$$

Where:
- Y is the dependent variable
- β_0 is the intercept (constant)
- $\beta_1, \beta_2, ..., \beta_n$ are the coefficients of the independent variables
- $X_1, X_2, ..., X_n$ are the independent variables
- ε is the error term

Applications of Regression

Prediction of Surgical Outcomes

Regression analysis is employed to predict surgical outcomes based on preoperative and intraoperative variables. For instance, Li et al. (2025-02-10) utilized regression analysis to classify and correlate orbital medial wall fractures with computed tomography data, aiding in the prediction of surgical planning. This helps surgeons to anticipate the complexity of the surgery and plan accordingly.

Assessing the Impact of Environmental Factors

Environmental factors, such as secondhand smoke (SHS) exposure, have been studied for their impact on eye health. Lu et al. (2025-02-11) demonstrated that regression analysis could establish the association between SHS exposure and an increased risk of developing myopia among nonmyopic children in China. By identifying these relationships, public health interventions can be designed to mitigate such risks.

Correlation of Clinical Features and Imaging Data

Regression analysis is also utilized to correlate clinical features with imaging data. Nguyen et al. (June 2012) explored the correlation between optical coherence tomography (OCT)-derived assessments of lower tear meniscus parameters and clinical features of dry eye disease. This analysis helps in understanding how clinical symptoms relate to imaging findings, thereby enhancing diagnostic accuracy and treatment planning.

Understanding Disease Mechanisms

By analyzing the relationship between various clinical and biological variables, regression analysis can unravel the underlying mechanisms of diseases. For example, Pan et al. (2025 Feb 11) studied the effect of modified surgical conditions on the peripapillary microvasculature and retinal nerve fiber layer (RNFL) in patients undergoing vitrectomy. The regression analysis provided insights into how surgical modifications could influence these ocular structures, contributing to better surgical techniques and patient outcomes.

■ CONCLUSION

In summary, regression analysis serves as a powerful tool in ophthalmology, facilitating the exploration of intricate relationships between clinical features, imaging data, and systemic factors. By employing these analytical techniques, researchers and clinicians can gain deeper insights into disease mechanisms, enhance diagnostic precision, and improve therapeutic strategies. The studies highlighted in this chapter underscore the importance of integrating statistical methods in medical research, ultimately aiming for better patient outcomes and advancing the field of ophthalmology.

■ BIBLIOGRAPHY

1. Li B, Feng L, Tang H, Wang F, Lin W, Classification and correlation analysis of orbital medial wall fractures based on computed tomography data for prediction of surgical planning. BMC Ophthalmology [Internet]. 2025 (cited 2025-02-10); 25(1). Available from: https://doi.org/10.1186/s12886-025-03900-8
2. Li D, Wang Q. Correlation analysis between nerve fiber layer thickness and peripapillary vessel density and influencing factors of peripapillary vessel density in preclinical diabetic retinopathy. J Ophthalmol [Internet]. 2020 (cited 2020/01/01);2020(1). Available from: https://doi.org/10.1155/2020/2758547
3. Lin H-Y, Wu W-C, Sun M-H, Lin J-Y, Huang P-H, Liu C-H. Measurements of objective cyclotorsion in a population of healthy children. J Ophthalmol [Internet]. 2024 (cited 2024/01/01);2024(1). Available from: https://doi.org/10.1155/joph/6982201
4. Lu Y, Li X, Deng Y, Wang K, Li Y, Zhao M. Secondhand smoke (SHS) exposure is associated with an increased risk of developing myopia among nonmyopic children in China. BMC Ophthalmology [Internet]. 2025 (cited 2025-02-11);25(1). Available from: https://doi.org/10.1186/s12886-025-03890-7
5. Martin J, Bradley C, Kran BS, Ross NC. Frontiers | Rasch analysis and targeting assessment of the teach-CVI survey tool in a cohort of CVI patients. Front Ophthalmol [Internet]. 2024 (cited 2024/11/29);4. Available from: https://doi.org/10.3389/fopht.2024.1495000
6. Nguyen DQ, Ross CM, Li YQ, Pandav S, Gardiner B, Smith D, et al. A model to measure fluid outflow in rabbit capsules post glaucoma implant surgery. Invest

Ophthalmol Vis Sci [Internet]. 2012 (cited 2012);53(11):6914-19. Available from: https://doi.org/10.1167/iovs.12-10438
7. Pan T, Bian C, Fang Y, Wang J, Xu Y, Xie P, et al. Effect of modified surgical conditions on the peripapillary microvasculature and RNFL in patients receiving vitrectomy: an OCTA study. BMC Ophthalmology [Internet]. 2025 (cited 2025/02/11);25(1). Available from: https://doi.org/10.1186/s12886-024-03832-9
8. Wang D, Marous C, Celiker P, Deng W, Kristoferson E, Elsayed A, et al. Frontiers | The association of race with thyroid eye disease presentation and outcomes. Front Ophthalmol [Internet]. 2024 (cited 2024/01/23);3.Available from: https://doi.org/10.3389/fopht.2023.1309850

CHAPTER 10

Inferential Statistics

T Raveendra, Annaji Rao Kota, Durga Bhavani Mummina

■ INTRODUCTION

In the vast and intricate realm of statistics, inferential statistics stand out as a profoundly powerful tool that empowers researchers, including ophthalmologists, to move beyond mere data collection and description. By delving into this chapter, you will embark on a comprehensive journey to uncover the methodologies and principles that allow for the analysis of data samples to make informed predictions and draw insightful inferences about larger populations, particularly in the field of eye health.

Inferential statistics enable ophthalmologists to understand the reliability of their research results, providing mechanisms to generalize findings beyond the immediate data at hand. This branch of statistics is essential for several key purposes, including:

- *Hypothesis testing:* Assessing hypotheses about population parameters based on sample data, such as determining the effectiveness of new treatments for eye diseases.
- *Determining probability:* Evaluating the likelihood that observed differences between treatment groups are due to random chance rather than the actual intervention.
- *Estimating population parameters:* Using sample data to estimate numerical characteristics of the entire population, such as the prevalence of certain eye conditions.

Techniques such as confidence intervals and *p*-values are integral to inferential statistics, enabling ophthalmologists to make decisions and draw conclusions with a certain level of confidence. Confidence intervals provide a range of values within which the true population parameter is likely to fall, while *p*-values help to determine the statistical significance of the results.

Essentially, inferential statistics allow for generalizations that extend beyond the immediate dataset, offering profound insights into broader trends and relationships within the population. This chapter will equip ophthalmologists with the knowledge and tools to navigate and apply these techniques effectively, enhancing their ability to make data-driven decisions and contribute meaningfully to the advancement of eye care and treatment.

In addition to these fundamental techniques, this chapter will also delve into the application of sensitivity and specificity, two critical concepts in medical statistics that are particularly vital for ophthalmologists when dealing with practical application of investigations for diagnosis. Sensitivity, or the true positive rate, measures the proportion of actual positives correctly identified by a diagnostic test, such as identifying patients with a particular eye disease. Specificity, or the true negative rate, assesses the proportion of actual negatives correctly identified, ensuring that healthy individuals are not misdiagnosed.

These concepts are closely related to *p*-values; in that, they help quantify the accuracy and reliability of diagnostic tests. By understanding and applying sensitivity and specificity, ophthalmologists can enhance their ability to evaluate the performance of new diagnostic tools and treatments, ultimately improving patient care and outcomes.

■ ESSENTIAL CONCEPTS

Inferential statistics involve using data from a sample to make inferences or predictions about a population. This branch of statistics is essential for hypothesis testing, determining the probability that an observed difference between groups is due to chance, and estimating population parameters. Techniques such as confidence intervals and *p*-values come into play, enabling researchers to make decisions and draw conclusions with a certain level of confidence. Essentially, inferential statistics allow for generalizations beyond the immediate data, providing insight into broader trends and relationships within the population.

Population

In statistics, a *population* refers to the entire set of individuals, items, or data points that share a common characteristic and are of interest in a particular study.

Sample

Sample is a subset of individuals, items, or data points selected from a larger population. The sample is used to make inferences about the population because it is often impractical or impossible to study the entire population. By analyzing the sample, researchers can estimate population parameters and draw conclusions about the population as a whole.

Parameter

A *parameter* is a numerical value that describes a specific characteristic of a population. It is a fixed value, though it is often unknown and estimated using sample data. Parameters provide a summary measure of the entire population and are used in statistical analysis to make inferences about the population. Examples are mean, standard deviation, variance, median, and mode.

Statistic

Statistic is a numerical characteristic of a sample, and used to estimate the corresponding parameter in the population.

Degrees of Freedom

Degrees of freedom represent the number of values in a calculation that are free to vary while estimating a statistical parameter.

Examples:
For a chi-square goodness of fit test, the degrees of freedom is k-1.

When estimating the mean of a single sample, the degrees of freedom is n – 1.

In ANOVA, degrees of freedom are calculated for both the between-group and within-group variations:
- Between-group degrees of freedom: df between = k – 1
- Within-group degrees of freedom: df within = n – k

Hypothesis Testing

Hypothesis testing is particularly useful in ophthalmology, where researchers and clinicians frequently seek to determine the efficacy of treatments, the progression of diseases, and the impact of various interventions on eye health. By employing hypothesis testing, ophthalmologists can make informed decisions based on empirical data, ultimately improving patient care and outcomes.

Hypothesis testing involves several key steps:
- *Formulating the hypotheses:* This includes the null hypothesis (H0), which states there is no effect or difference, and the alternative hypothesis (H1), which states there is a significant effect or difference.
- *Selecting the significance level:* Commonly denoted as alpha (α), this is the threshold for determining whether to reject the null hypothesis. The typical value is 0.05.
- *Choosing the test statistic:* Depending on the type of data and the hypothesis, this could be a t-test, Chi-square test, ANOVA, etc.
- *Calculating the test statistic and p-value:* The test statistic helps determine how far the sample data deviates from the null hypothesis. The *p*-value indicates the probability of obtaining the observed results if the null hypothesis is true.
- *Making a decision:* If the *p*-value is less than the significance level (α), the null hypothesis is rejected in favor of the alternative hypothesis. Otherwise, we fail to reject the null hypothesis.

Here is an example relevant to ophthalmology:
- *Example hypothesis:* The average intraocular pressure (IOP) in patients treated with drug A is the same as in those treated with drug B.
- *Null hypothesis (H0):* The mean IOP for drug A equals the mean IOP for drug B.
- *Alternative hypothesis (H1):* The mean IOP for drug A does not equal the mean IOP for drug B.
- *Significance level (α):* 0.05
- *Test statistic*: A t-test for comparing two means can be used.
- *Calculate and decision:* Based on the sample data, calculate the t-test statistic and corresponding p-value. If p-value < 0.05, reject H0, indicating a significant difference in IOP between drug A and drug B.

In summary, hypothesis testing provides a structured framework for making data-driven decisions in ophthalmology, ensuring that conclusions about treatments and interventions are based on robust statistical evidence.

Hypothesis testing is a statistical method used to make decisions or inferences about a population based on sample data. It involves testing an assumption (the hypothesis) about a population parameter. It is commonly employed to assess the significance of results.

Null Hypothesis

In the realm of statistics, the null hypothesis is a fundamental concept that serves as the starting point for hypothesis testing. Essentially, it is a statement suggesting that there is no effect, no difference, or no relationship between variables in a given population. The null hypothesis, often denoted as H_0, assumes that any observed differences in data are attributable to random chance rather than being caused by a specific factor or intervention.

It serves as a default or baseline assumption that any observed differences or effects are due to random chance or variability rather than a specific cause or intervention.

Examples:
- The average IOP between patients treated with drug A and drug B is equal.
- There is no significant difference in the rate of progression of diabetic retinopathy between patients on a low-sugar diet and those on a regular diet.
- The mean retinal thickness in patients with macular edema
- Is the same before and after treatment with the new medication
- There is no significant difference in the incidence of cataracts between patients exposed to ultraviolet (UV) light and those who are not.
- The average recovery time after cataract surgery is the same for patients using two different types of intraocular lenses.

- There is no association between the duration of diabetes and the severity of diabetic retinopathy.
- The prevalence of dry eye syndrome is equal among contact lens wearers and nonwearers.
- There is no significant difference in the visual field loss between patients with open-angle glaucoma and those with angle-closure glaucoma.

Alternative Hypothesis

An *alternative hypothesis* (denoted as H1 or HA) is a statement in statistical hypothesis testing that proposes there is a significant effect or difference between groups or variables. It is the hypothesis that researchers aim to support through their study. The alternative hypothesis is contrasted with the null hypothesis (H0), which suggests that there is no effect or difference.

The alternative hypothesis can be one-sided (directional) or two-sided (nondirectional):
- *One-sided alternative hypothesis:* Specifies the direction of the effect (e.g., "the new drug lowers blood pressure")
- *Two-sided alternative hypothesis:* Does not specify the direction, only that there is a difference (e.g., "the new drug affects blood pressure")

For example, in a study examining the effect of a new drug on blood pressure, the hypotheses might be:
- *Null hypothesis (H0):* The new drug has no effect on blood pressure.
- *Alternative hypothesis (H1):* The new drug affects blood pressure (two-sided)
  (or)
  The new drug lowers blood pressure (one-sided).

The goal of hypothesis testing is to determine whether there is enough evidence to reject the null hypothesis in favor of the alternative hypothesis.

Examples:
- The average IOP between patients treated with drug A and drug B is different.
- There is a significant difference in the rate of progression of diabetic retinopathy between patients on a low-sugar diet and those on a regular diet.
- The mean retinal thickness in patients with macular edema is different before and after treatment with the new medication.
- There is a significant difference in the incidence of cataracts between patients exposed to UV light and those who are not.
- The average recovery time after cataract surgery is different for patients using two different types of intraocular lenses.

- There is an association between the duration of diabetes and the severity of diabetic retinopathy.
- The prevalence of dry eye syndrome is different among contact lens wearers and nonwearers.
- There is a significant difference in the visual field loss between patients with open-angle glaucoma and those with angle-closure glaucoma.

Confidence Interval

A confidence interval offers a range of values where the true population parameter is likely to be found, with a specified level of confidence. For instance, a 95% confidence interval for the population mean suggests that we are 95% certain the true mean lies within this range. Confidence intervals help measure the uncertainty in model predictions or parameter estimates.

Confidence intervals are especially useful in ophthalmology research because they provide a range within which we can be reasonably confident that the true effect size lies. This is vital when evaluating the effectiveness of treatments or interventions for eye diseases.

For example, in a study comparing two types of intraocular lenses, a 95% confidence interval for the difference in average recovery times might range from 2–5 days. This suggests that we are 95% confident that the true difference in recovery times falls within this interval, offering valuable insight into the potential benefits of one lens over the other.

Moreover, confidence intervals help assess the precision of estimated differences in clinical outcomes. For instance, when measuring changes in retinal thickness before and after treatment for macular edema, a narrower confidence interval indicates more precise estimates, thereby providing stronger evidence for the treatment's effectiveness.

In addition to providing estimates for treatment effects, confidence intervals allow ophthalmologists to gauge the reliability of diagnostic tests. For instance, in determining the sensitivity and specificity of a new diagnostic tool for detecting glaucoma, confidence intervals give a range for these parameters, helping clinicians understand the test's accuracy and potential limitations.

Furthermore, confidence intervals aid in the interpretation of the clinical significance of study results. While a statistically significant *p*-value indicates that an observed effect is unlikely to be due to chance, the confidence interval provides context for the magnitude and clinical relevance of the effect.

Ultimately, confidence intervals are an indispensable tool for ophthalmologists, enabling them to make informed decisions based on both the statistical and clinical significance of their research findings.

Sensitivity–Specificity and Likelihood Ratios

Sensitivity and specificity are pivotal metrics in evaluating the performance of diagnostic tests in ophthalmology. Sensitivity, also known as the true positive rate, measures the proportion of actual positives correctly identified by the test. For instance, in assessing a new diagnostic tool for glaucoma, a high sensitivity rate indicates that the test is adept at identifying patients with the condition, minimizing the risk of false negatives.

Specificity, on the other hand, is the true negative rate, representing the proportion of actual negatives accurately identified. In the same glaucoma diagnostic context, high specificity means that the test effectively recognizes patients without the condition, reducing the likelihood of false positives. Sensitivity and specificity together measure a test's diagnostic accuracy. They are used to calculate likelihood ratios (LRs), which help determine how much a test result will change the probability of having a disease.

Concept of Likelihood Ratios

Likelihood ratios offer a nuanced interpretation of diagnostic tests by combining sensitivity and specificity into a single measure. The positive likelihood ratio (LR^+) indicates how much the odds of the disease increase when a test is positive, whereas the negative likelihood ratio (LR^-) shows how much the odds decrease when a test is negative. LRs are instrumental in refining clinical judgment, particularly when pretest probabilities of disease are considered.

For example, in the case of diabetic retinopathy, an ophthalmologist may use an LR^+ to assess how a positive test result shifts the probability of a patient having the disease. Conversely, an LR– helps determine how a negative result impacts the likelihood of the disease. By integrating sensitivity, specificity, and LRs, ophthalmologists can make more informed decisions, ensuring accurate diagnoses and effective patient care.

Pre and Post-test Probabilities

To transition from LRs to probabilities in diagnosis, clinicians often use tools like the Fagan nomogram or apply Bayes' theorem. The process typically involves three key steps:
1. *Pretest probability*: Assess the pretest probability of the disease, which is the clinician's initial estimation of the likelihood that the disease is present before conducting the test. This assessment can be based on clinical judgment, patient history, prevalence data, or other relevant factors.

2. *Likelihood ratios:* Use the test's LRs—the LR+ and the LR. The LR+ is applied when the test result is positive, and the LR− is applied when the test result is negative. These ratios indicate how much the test result will alter the odds of having the disease.
3. *Post-test probability:* Convert the pretest probability to odds, apply the LR, and then convert the post-test odds back to probability. This conversion can be performed mathematically or graphically using the Fagan nomogram.

Mathematically, the steps are as follows:
- *Convert the pretest probability (P) to pretest odds*: Odds = $P/(1 − P)$
- Multiply the pretest odds by the LR to get the post-test odds.
- *Convert the post-test odds back to probability*: Probability = Odds/(1 + Odds).

For example, if an ophthalmologist suspects diabetic retinopathy and estimates a pretest probability of 30% (0.30), the pretest odds would be $0.30/(1 − 0.30) = 0.43$. If the test has an LR^+ of 5, the post-test odds would be $0.43 \times 5 = 2.15$. Converting these odds back to probability gives $2.15/(1 + 2.15) \approx 0.68$, or 68%. Thus, a positive test result significantly increases the likelihood of the disease.

p-value

In the realm of ophthalmology, where precision and accuracy are paramount, the *p*-value stands as a crucial metric. It quantifies the evidence against the null hypothesis, serving as a beacon for researchers navigating the complexities of clinical trial results. When investigating the efficacy of new treatments for conditions such as diabetic retinopathy or glaucoma, understanding the *p*-value allows ophthalmologists to determine the statistical significance of their findings.

The *p*-value indicates the strength of the evidence against the null hypothesis. A smaller *p*-value (e.g., <0.05) suggests strong evidence to reject the null hypothesis, while a larger *p*-value indicates insufficient evidence to do so.

Significance Level (α)

The significance level (α) is a critical concept in statistical hypothesis testing. It represents the probability of making a Type I Error, which is rejecting a true null hypothesis. By setting a significance level, researchers define the threshold at which they will consider the results statistically significant. Commonly used significance levels are 0.05, 0.01, and 0.10. For example, a significance level of 0.05 implies that there is a 5% chance of rejecting the null hypothesis when it is actually true.

A threshold set by the researcher which the *p*-value must be below in order to reject the null hypothesis. Commonly used significance levels are 0.05, 0.01, and 0.10.

Type I Error

The error made when a true null hypothesis is incorrectly rejected.

Type II Error

The error made when a false null hypothesis is not rejected.

True positive, false positives, false negatives, and true negatives.

In the field of ophthalmology, understanding Type I and Type II errors is critical for the interpretation of clinical trial results and the evaluation of new treatments.

Type I error (false positive) occurs when an ophthalmologist incorrectly concludes that treatment is effective when it is not. For instance, a new eye drop may appear to improve IOP in clinical trials due to random chance rather than its actual efficacy. This can lead to the premature adoption of ineffective treatments, exposing patients to unnecessary side effects or delaying access to better therapies.

Type II error (false negative) happens when an ophthalmologist fails to detect a true effect of a treatment, such as overlooking the benefits of a new surgical technique for glaucoma. This might occur due to insufficient sample size or variability in patient responses. Missing a genuinely effective treatment means that valuable therapeutic advancements are not recognized or implemented, potentially impacting patient outcomes.

■ PARAMETRIC TESTS

Parametric tests are statistical tests that assume the data follows a certain distribution, typically a normal distribution. They are powerful tools for hypothesis testing and can provide more precise estimates when the assumptions are met. These tests are particularly useful in ophthalmology research, where precise measurements and robust data are often available **(Flowchart 10.1)**.

Common parametric tests include the t-test, which compares the meanings of two groups, and analysis of variance (ANOVA), which compares the means of three or more groups. These tests rely on parameters such as the mean and standard deviation, offering a detailed understanding of the data's underlying structure.

In the realm of ophthalmology, parametric tests can be used to evaluate the efficacy of new treatments, compare visual acuity outcomes, or analyze IOP variations among different patient groups. Ensuring that the data meets the assumptions of normality and homogeneity of variance is crucial for the validity of these tests.

Chi-square Test

The Chi-square test is one of the most common tests applicable in various specialties, especially when dealing with categorical data. It assesses the association between two variables by comparing the observed frequencies with the expected frequencies under the null hypothesis of no association. However, a prerequisite for the selection of this test is the normality of the distribution of data. If the data does not follow normal distribution, alternative tests must be considered.

Chi-square Test of Independence

Another common use of the Chi-square test is to determine whether one or more attributes are associated. In the previous section, we used one-way classification tables of observed frequencies in a single row or column. When individuals can be classified in two different ways, forming rows and columns, the resulting table is called a contingency table. It is sometimes desirable to compare one set of observations taken under specific conditions with a similar set taken under different conditions. In this case, there are no expected values, and the question is whether the results are dependent on or independent of the conditions under which they occurred. This test is known as the test for independence or the contingency test.

Characteristics of Chi-square Test

- This test is based on frequencies, whereas, in theoretical distribution, the test is based on mean and standard deviation.
- The other distribution can be used for testing the significance of the difference between a single expected value and observed proportion. However, this test can be used for testing difference between the entire set of the expected and the observed frequencies.
- A new Chi-square distribution is formed for every increase in the number of degrees of freedom.
- This test is applied for testing the hypothesis but is not useful for estimation.

Assumptions of Validity of Chi-square Test

- All the observations must be independent. No individual item should be included twice or a number of times in the sample.
- The total number of observations should be large. The Chi-square test should be used if $n > 50$.
- All the events must be mutually exclusive.
- For comparison purposes, the data must be in original units.
- If the theoretical frequency is <5, then we pool it with the preceding or the succeeding frequency, so that the resulting sim is >5.

Applications of Chi-square Test

The Chi-square test is a valuable tool in various fields such as agriculture, biology, medical sciences, and other statistical analyses. Its main applications include:

Testing the independence of attributes: This application helps determine if two categorical variables are related or independent from each other. The Chi-square test can also be used in ophthalmology to determine if there is an association between contact lens usage and the incidence of eye infections. By comparing the observed frequency of infections in contact lens users versus nonusers against expected frequencies, researchers can assess if there is a significant relationship between these variables.

For example, in biology, researchers can use it to analyze if certain genetic traits are associated with specific populations.

Testing goodness of fit: This application assesses how well-observed data conforms to an expected distribution. For instance, in medical sciences, it can be applied to see if a sample of patient recovery times follows a normal distribution. Similarly, in biology, it can check if the frequency of different species in a region matches expected proportions based on past data.

These applications enable researchers to draw meaningful conclusions and make informed decisions based on statistical evidence as illustrated in **(Tables 10.1a and 10.1b)**.

Comparison of Means of Two Variables (t-test)

A *t-test* is a statistical test used to compare the means of two groups and determine whether the differences between them are statistically significant. It is commonly used when the sample sizes are small and the population variance is unknown. There are several types of t-tests, each suited for different scenarios **(Table 10.2)**.

TABLE 10.1(a): Table depicting patient satisfaction after laser in situ keratomileusis in myopic patients.

Relation between satisfaction and age, sex, residence, occupation, degree of myopia, and previous glasses of the studied patients

		Totally unsatisfied (n = 2)	Mild unsatisfaction (n = 12)	Neutral (n = 26)	Mild satisfaction (n = 26)	Totally satisfied (n = 34)	p
Age (years)		38 ± 1.41	34.3 ± 5.57	28.9 ± 6.54	29.8 ± 5.32	28.9 ± 4.79	0.009
	P1		0.906	0.169	0.257	0.159	
	P2			0.043	0.131	0.031	
	P3				0.978	1	
	P4					0.968	
Sex	Male	2 (100%)	9 (75%)	20 (76.92%)	14 (53.85%)	6 (17.65%)	<0.001
	Female	0 (0%)	3 (25%)	6 (23.08%)	12 (46.15%)	28 (82.35%)	
Residency	Urban	2 (100%)	9 (75%)	16 (61.54%)	19 (73.08%)	17 (50%)	<0.001
	Rural	0 (0%)	3 (25%)	10 (38.46%)	7 (26.92%)	17 (50%)	
Occupation	Engineer	0 (0%)	2 (16.67%)	2 (7.69%)	2 (7.69%)	1 (2.94%)	0.091
	Accountant	0 (0%)	3 (25%)	2 (7.69%)	2 (7.69%)	3 (8.82%)	
	Housewife	0 (0%)	1 (8.33%)	0 (0%)	4 (15.38%)	11 (32.35%)	
	Pharmacist	0 (0%)	0 (0%)	1 (3.85%)	1 (3.85%)	1 (2.94%)	
	Doctor	1 (50%)	0 (0%)	2 (7.69%)	3 (11.54%)	4 (11.76%)	
	Teacher	0 (0%)	0 (0%)	1 (3.85%)	0 (0%)	2 (5.88%)	
	Student	0 (0%)	0 (0%)	4 (15.38%)	2 (7.69%)	3 (8.82%)	
	Driver	0 (0%)	0 (0%)	5 (19.23%)	1 (3.85%)	0 (0%)	

Contd...

Contd...

	Totally unsatisfied (n = 2)	Mild unsatisfaction (n = 12)	Neutral (n = 26)	Mild satisfaction (n = 26)	Totally satisfied (n = 34)	p
Physical therapy	0 (0%)	0 (0%)		0 (0%)	1 (2.94%)	
Police officer	0 (0%)	0 (0%)	1 (3.85%)	1 (3.85%)	1 (2.94%)	
Worker	0 (0%)	1 (8.33%)	1 (3.85%)	2 (7.69%)	5 (14.71%)	
Judge	0 (0%)	1 (8.33%)	1 (3.85%)	2 (7.69%)	0 (0%)	
Football player	0 (0%)	0 (0%)	1 (3.85%)	0 (0%)	0 (0%)	
Farmer	0 (0%)	0 (0%)	2 (7.69%)	0 (0%)	0 (0%)	
Seller	0 (0%)	0 (0%)	1 (3.85%)	0 (0%)	0 (0%)	
Technician	1 (50%)	1 (8.33%)	1 (3.85%)	1 (3.85%)	0 (0%)	
Assistant lecturer	0 (0%)	0 (0%)	0 (0%)	1 (3.85%)	0 (0%)	
Nurse	0 (0%)	1 (8.33%)	0 (0%)	4 (15.38%)	0 (0%)	
Lawyer	0 (0%)	0 (0%)	0 (0%)	0 (0%)	2 (5.88%)	
Translator	0 (0%)	0 (0%)	1 (3.85%)	0 (0%)	0 (0%)	
Dentist	0 (0%)	1 (8.33%)	0 (0%)	0 (0%)	0 (0%)	
Barbar	0 (0%)	1 (8.33%)	0 (0%)	0 (0%)	0 (0%)	
Previous glasses	2 (100%)	7 (58.33%)	13 (50%)	14 (53.85%)	9 (26.47%)	0.058
Degree of myopia	3.1 ± 1.94	3.3 ± 1.91	3.1 ± 1.68	3.5 ± 1.75	3.6 ± 1.56	0.775

TABLE 10.1b: Explanation for the above **Table 10.1a** depicting application of patient satisfaction after laser in situ keratomileusis in myopic patients.

The tabulation representing proportions for various categories needs to be assessed for significances. The modalities in selection of significance depends also on *degrees of freedom represented by number of rows—1 and number of columns—1 which is taken care by statisticians.*	
Chi-square test and other test used in table to be checked from article reference	Where the data are qualitative and in proportions, and multiple rows, the Chi-square test has been applied for *p*-value For instances where the data are qualitative and measured in proportions across multiple rows, the Chi-Square test has been utilized to determine the P-Value. For single row data, as illustrated by "Previous Glasses" and "Degree of Myopia", the appropriate statistical test applied is a Fisher's Exact Test

TABLE 10.2: Overview of t-tests.

Test type	Description	Steps to perform	Null hypothesis (H0)	Alternative hypothesis (H1)
Paired t-test	Compares the means of two related groups, suitable for nonindependent samples	Formulate hypotheses	The mean difference between paired observations is zero	The mean difference between paired observations is not zero
Independent t-test	Compares the means of two unrelated groups, used for independent samples	Formulate hypotheses	The means of the two groups are equal	The means of the two groups are not equal

Comparison of Sets of Independent Data: Independence t-test

An *independent t-test* (also known as a two-sample t-test or unpaired t-test) is a statistical test used to compare the means of two independent groups to determine whether there is a statistically significant difference between them. This test is commonly used when the two groups are not related or paired in any way **[Tables 10.3(a) and 10.3(b)]**.

TABLE 10.3a: Table depicting effect of intravitreal antivascular endothelial growth factor injection in corneal thickness.

Comparison of preinjection and postinjection (day 1, 7, and 30) CCT (µm) between pseudophakic and phakic group			
Parameter	Group 2 pseudophakic	Group 1 phakic	P (intergroup)
Preinjection CCT	503.9 ± 19.1	506.5 ± 22.6 (−0.07% ± 2.08%)	0.632
CCT day 1	502.0 ± 19.9 (0.34% ± 3.03%)	505.9 ± 20.1 (−0.07% ± 2.60%)	0.328
CCT day 7	501.9 ± 20.3 (−0.36% ± 3.46%)	505.9 ± 20.3	0.298
CCT day 30	501.7 ± 21.5 (0.40% ± 3.65%)	505.6 ± 21.4 (−0.12% ± 2.60%)	0.416

TABLE 10.3b: Explanation for the above **Table 10.3a** depicting effect of intravitreal antivascular endothelial growth.

In a study "effect of intravitreal antivascular endothelial growth factor on corneal endothelial cell count and central corneal thickness in Indian population"	
Importance of independent t-test	• Independent t-test is applicable to compare the averages between the two independent groups • Phakic eyes are those with a natural lens, whereas pseudophakic eyes have had the natural lens replaced with an artificial one, usually due to cataract surgery. When assessing the impact of intravitreal anti-VEGF injections on corneal endothelial cell count and central corneal thickness, it is important to distinguish between these two types of eyes because their anatomical and physiological differences can influence the treatment's effects independently. Thus, they are considered separately to ensure accurate evaluation and results. • The other t-test is paired t-test
(VEGF: vascular endothelial growth factor)	

Independent groups: The two groups being compared are separate and do not influence each other. For example, comparing the test scores of students from two different schools.

Assumptions:
- The data in each group are normally distributed.
- The variances of the two groups are equal (homogeneity of variance).
- The samples are independent of each other.

Steps to perform an independent t-test:
1. *Formulate hypotheses:*
   - *Null hypothesis (H_0):* The means of the two groups are equal ($\mu 1 = \mu 2$).
   - *Alternative hypothesis (H_1):* The means of the two groups are not equal.

2. *Choose the significance level (α):*
   - Common choices are 0.05, 0.01, or 0.10
3. *Calculate the test statistic:*
   The test statistic is calculated using the formula:

$$t = \frac{\bar{x}_1 - \bar{x}_2}{\sqrt{\frac{s_1^2}{n_1} + \frac{s_2^2}{n_2}}} \sim (n_1 + n_2 - 2)$$

Find the p-value: Using the t-distribution table, find the *p*-value corresponding to the calculated test statistic and degrees of freedom.

Interpretation: Compare the *p*-value to the significance level (α). If the *p*-value is less than or equal to α, reject the null hypothesis. If the *p*-value is greater than α, fail to reject the null hypothesis.

Comparison of Paired Data: Paired t-test

The *paired t-test* (also known as the dependent t-test) is a statistical test used to compare the means of two related groups. It is commonly used when the same subjects are measured twice under different conditions, or when there are matched pairs of subjects. The paired t-test helps determine whether the mean difference between the paired observations is statistically significant **[Tables 10.4(a) and 10.4(b)]**.

Steps to perform a paired t-test:
1. Formulate hypotheses:
   - *Null hypothesis (H0):* The mean difference between the paired observations is zero ($\mu d = 0$).
   - *Alternative hypothesis (H1):* The mean difference between the paired observations is not zero ($\mu d \neq 0$).
2. Calculate the difference scores:
   - For each pair, calculate the difference (d_i) between the two observations.
3. *Compute the mean and standard deviation of the difference scores:*
   - Calculate the mean difference ($\bar{d}$) and the standard deviation of the differences (S_d).
4. *Calculate the test statistic:* The test statistic is calculated using the formula:

$$t = \frac{\bar{d}}{S_d / \sqrt{n}}$$

5. *Determine the degrees of freedom (df):* The degrees of freedom for the paired t-test is $n - 1$, where n is the number of pairs.
6. *Find the p-value:* Using the t-distribution table, find the *p*-value corresponding to the calculated test statistic and degrees of freedom.

TABLE 10.4(a): Illustration for application of Paired t-test.

RNFL data from initial and final OCTs as well as disc area and rim area measured by OCT in eyes categorized as glaucoma suspects, on drops, or diagnosed with glaucoma at the time of final follow-up

		Glaucoma suspects	Drops	Glaucoma
Average RNFL (μm)	Initial	90.7 ± 16.8 (n = 49)	76 ± 17 (n = 2)	88.5 ± 0.7 (n = 2)
	Final	92.3 ± 13.5 (n = 88)	78.4 ± 9.1 (n = 5)	62 ± 4.2 (n = 2)
	p-value	0.5	0.8	0.01*
Inferior RNFL (μm)	Initial	113.5 ± 26.8 (n = 49)	103.5 ± 27.6 (n = 2)	102.5 ± 0.7 (n = 2)
	Final	120.9 ± 22.1 (n = 88)	108 ± 19.8 (n = 5)	71 ± 5.7 (n = 2)
	p-value	0.9	0.8	0.02*
Superior RNFL (μm)	Initial	118.1 ± 22.5 (n = 49)	86 ± 17 (n = 2)	118.5 ± 4.9 (n = 2)
	Final	114.4 ± 20.9 (n = 88)	96.8 ± 16.2 (n = 5)	59 ± 14.1 (n = 2)
	p-value	0.3	0.5	0.03*
Disc area (mm^2)		2.5 ± 0.5 (n = 106)	1.9 ± 0.4 (n = 7)	2.5 ± 0.6 (n = 4)
Rim area (mm^2)		1.3 ± 0.1 (n = 106)	1.3 ± 0.3 (n = 7)	1.4 ± 0.3 (n = 4)

Note: Significant findings are classified as $p \leq 0.05$ and are denoted with "*".
(RNFL: retinal nerve fiber layer)

TABLE 10.4(b): Explanation for the illustration in **Table 10.4(a)**, paired t-test applied for multiple groups, initial presentation and final follow-up.

In the above illustrated study titled as "Cup-to-disc ratio measured clinically and via OCT in pediatric patients being monitored as glaucoma suspects for suspicious optic discs"	
Importance of paired t-test	• Paired t-test can be applied for the related data to check the significancy for the averages for the two related groups. • In this particular study, paired t-test has been applied individually to all the above-mentioned three groups namely glaucoma suspects, dropouts, glaucoma cases at the time of presentation, and at 5 years of follow-up after initiation of antiglaucoma medication therapy. Here, we see that when comparing RNFL thickness in the first two groups, p-value >0.05 hence not significant but in the glaucoma group, p-value <0.05 hence significant
(OCT: optical coherence tomography; RNFL: retinal nerve fiber layer)	

7. *Interpretation:* Compare the p-value to the significance level (α). If the p-value is less than or equal to α, reject the null hypothesis. If the p-value is greater than α, fail to reject the null hypothesis.

Comparison of Means of Three or More Variables (F-test)

The F-test is a statistical method used to compare the variances of two or more groups to determine if they come from populations with equal variances. It is particularly useful in testing the hypothesis that the means of three or more groups are equal, which is essential in ANOVA (analysis of variance). By analyzing the ratio of the variance between the groups to the variance within the groups, the F-test helps identify if there are any significant differences among the group means.

Analysis of Variance

In the previous discussion, we explained how to compare the means of two samples using the t-test, which determines the significance of the difference between two means. However, we did not address the case of testing the significance of more than two sample means. In this section, we will focus on comparing the means of three or more samples, including the variations within each sample. When comparing more than two experimental or field samples, statistical techniques are used to test the homogeneity of means and the hypothesis that the means do not differ significantly. This statistical method, developed by RA Fisher, has been extensively used in agricultural experiments.

Types of ANOVA:
- One-way ANOVA
- Two-way ANOVA
- Repeated measures ANOVA

One-way ANOVA: One-way ANOVA (analysis of variance) is a statistical technique used to compare the means of three or more independent groups to determine if there is a statistically significant difference among them. It helps to understand if at least one group mean is different from the others **[Tables 10.5(a) and 10.5(b)]**.

Key concepts:
- *Independent variable (factor):* The categorical variable that divides the data into groups (e.g., different diets)
- *Dependent variable:* The continuous variable that you measure (e.g., weight loss)

Hypotheses:
- *Null hypothesis (H_0):* All group means are equal ($\mu 1 = \mu 2 = \mu 3 = \ldots = \mu k$)
- *Alternative hypothesis (H_1):* At least one group mean is different.

Assumptions:
- *Independence:* Observations in each group must be independent.
- *Normality:* The dependent variable should be approximately normally distributed within each group.
- *Homogeneity of variances:* The variances among the groups should be roughly equal.

Steps to perform one-way ANOVA:
- *Formulate hypotheses:* Define the null and alternative hypotheses.
- *Calculate ANOVA:*
  - *Between-group variance:* Measures the variation due to the interaction between the different groups.
  - *Within-group variance:* Measures the variation within each group.
  - *F-statistic:* The ratio of between-group variance to within-group variance.
- *Compare F-statistic:* Compare the calculated F-statistic to the critical value from the F-distribution table.
- *Interpret results:* If the F-statistic is greater than the critical value, reject the null hypothesis.

Illustrations:
- Imagine a researcher wants to compare the effectiveness of three different teaching methods on student performance. They would:
  - Collect test scores from students using each teaching method.

TABLE 10.5a: Illustration of the concept of ANOVA being applied to a study involving variants of ACE gene.

Clinical characteristics of groups of patients depending on the ACE gene variant.

Characteristic	Group 1 with ACE genotype II (n = 28)	Group 2 with ACE genotype ID (n = 47)	Group 3 with ACE genotype DD (n = 19)	p
Age (years)	63.5 (55–70)	64 (57.75–70)	61 (56.25–70.75)	0.831
Pulmonary parenchymal lesions, M±SD (%)	50.6 ± 15.5	50.9 ± 14.3	52.2 ± 17	0.934
Blood oxygen saturation level (%) (IQR)	92.5 (84–96.5)	92 (88.25–96)	93 (88.25–96.75)	0.851
Oxygen flow speed, L/min, used to maintain normal blood saturation (IQR)	11 (8–14.5)	12 (8–17.75)	10 (8.5–16)	0.726
SBP (IQR), mm Hg	130 (125–140)	130 (125–140)	130 (130–140)	0.396
DBP (IQR), mm Hg	80 (80–90)	80 (80–90)	80 (80–90)	0.695
Heart rate (M±SD), beats/min	91 ± 17.5	92.7 ± 16.2	90.7 ± 14.6	0.873
Respiratory rate, breaths/min M±SD	24.2 ± 4.4	24.3 ± 4.1	25.1 ± 4.7	0.765
D-dimer level (IQR), N, up to 0.5 μg/mL	0.66 (0.34–1.18)	0.79 (0.31–2.22)	1.09 (0.43–2.28)	0.380
Women (n, %)	16 (57.1)	25 (53.2)	11 (57.9)	0.916
Men (n, %)	12 (42.9)	22 (46.8)	8 (42.1)	
Comorbidity: type 1 or type 2 diabetes mellitus (n, %)	5 (17.9)	4 (8.5)	2 (10.5)	0.469
Comorbidity: hypertensive heart disease (n, %)	9 (32.1)	15 (31.9)	5 (26.3)	0.891

Note: DBP: diastolic blood pressure; N: norm; P: significance of difference; n: number; SBP: systolic blood pressure (ACE: angiotensin-converting enzyme; ANOVA: analysis of variance)

- Use one-way ANOVA to determine if there are significant differences in test scores between the teaching methods.
- If ANOVA shows significant differences, conduct post-hoc tests (e.g., Tukey's HSD) to identify which teaching methods differ.
  - Comparing central foveal thickness measurement in three intravitreal injection groups—bevacizumab, ranibizumab, and aflibercept.

Post-hoc tests: If the ANOVA indicates significant differences, post-hoc tests are used to determine which specific groups differ from each other. Common post-hoc tests include:
  - Tukey's HSD (honestly significant difference)
  - Bonferroni correction
  - Scheff's test

TABLE 10.5(b): Explanation for the above **Table 10.5(a)** depicting the content for ANOVA application

In the study mentioned, an ANOVA test was used to compare three different groups, based on genotype, to determine the correlation with the severity of COVID-19 infection. The results showed a p-value > 0.05 in all groups, indicating no statistical significance.	
Importance of ANOVA	• The ANOVA test is used to determine if there are any statistically significant differences between the means of three or more independent groups in a normally distributed data set • ANOVA allows for the comparison of multiple groups simultaneously, rather than conducting multiple t-tests, which increases the risk of Type I errors (false positives) • ANOVA helps in understanding the variability within and between groups as in this example, providing insights into the factors that may influence the outcome • By comparing all groups at once, ANOVA is more efficient and less time-consuming than performing multiple pairwise comparisons
(ANOVA: analysis of variance)	

Two-way ANOVA: Two-way ANOVA is used to determine how two factors (independent variables) influence a dependent variable and whether there is an interaction effect between the two factors **[Tables 10.6(a) and 10.6(b)]**.

Key concepts:
- *Factors:* The two independent variables being studied (e.g., diet and exercise)
- *Levels:* The different categories or groups within each factor (e.g., different types of diets and different exercise routines)
- *Interaction effect:* Occurs when the effect of one factor depends on the level of the other factor

TABLE 10.6(a): Study analyzing relation of axial length to corneal curvature radius ratio with choroidal.

ANOVA results of the mean axial, AL/CR, and macular fovea choroidal perfusion after grouping by myopia severity

		Sum of squares	Degree of freedom	Mean square	F	Significance
Axial Length In 3 Myopia severity groups	Between groups | 3 groups	88.802	2	44.401	84.309	<0.000
	Intra-group	104.803	199	0.527		
	Total	193.605	201			
AL/CR In 3 Myopia severity groups	Between groups | 3 groups	1.531	2	0.765	143.555	<0.000
	Intra-group	1.061	199	0.005		
	Total	2.591	201			
Macular foveal choroidal perfusion	Between groups | 3 groups	0.044	2	0.022	10.421	<0.000
	Intra-group	0.424	199	0.002		
	Total	0.468	201			

*Represents significance levels of 10% respectively.

TABLE 10.6(b): Explanation for the above **Table 10.6a**: Study analyzing relation of axial length to corneal curvature radius ratio with choroidal.

In the study analyzing relation of *axial length to corneal curvature radius ratio with choroidal blood flow in myopic children*	
Why is two-way ANOVA selected?	• Two-way ANOVA is selected in this study to examine the interaction of two independent variables: (1) The ratio of axial length to corneal curvature radius and (2) the choroidal blood flow • Both independently related factors are being studied for correlation • The result shows an inverse relationship, indicating that either could be primarily affecting the other in the inverse manner
(ANOVA: analysis of variance)	

Hypotheses:

Main effects:
- Null hypothesis (H_0): The means of the dependent variable are equal across the levels of each factor.
- Alternative hypothesis (H_1): At least one mean is different across the levels of each factor.

Interaction effect:
- Null hypothesis (H_0): There is no interaction effect between the two factors.
- Alternative hypothesis (H_1): There is an interaction effect between the two factors.

Assumptions:
- *Independence:* Observations must be independent.
- *Normality:* The dependent variable should be approximately normally distributed within each group.
- *Homogeneity of variances:* The variances among the groups should be roughly equal.

Steps to perform two-way ANOVA:
1. *Formulate hypotheses:* Define the null and alternative hypotheses for the main effects and interaction effect.
2. *Calculate ANOVA:*
   - Sum of squares (SS): Calculate the SS for each main effect, the interaction effect, and the error.
   - Degrees of freedom (df): Determine the degrees of freedom for each source of variation.
   - Mean squares (MS): Calculate the MS by dividing the SS by the corresponding degrees of freedom.

- *F-statistic:* Compute the F-statistic for each main effect and the interaction effect.
3. *Compare F-statistic:* Compare the calculated F-statistics to the critical values from the F-distribution table.
4. *Interpret results:* Determine if the main effects and interaction effect are significant.

Comparing central foveal thickness in three injection groups (bevacizumab, ranibizumab, and aflibercept) and also between males and females in these three groups. Here, we have two independent groups: type of injection and gender.

Repeated measures ANOVA: Repeated measures ANOVA is used to compare means across multiple measurements taken from the same subjects. It accounts for the correlation between measurements taken from the same individual, which is a key difference from other types of ANOVA **[Tables 10.7(a) and 10.7(b)]**.

Key concepts:
- *Within-subjects factor:* The independent variable that has multiple levels, with each level representing a different condition or time point (e.g., different treatments or time periods)
- *Dependent variable:* The continuous variable that you measure (e.g., blood pressure, test scores)

Hypotheses:
- *Null hypothesis (H_0):* The means of the dependent variable are equal across all levels of the within-subjects factor.
- *Alternative hypothesis (H_1):* At least one mean is different across the levels of the within-subjects factor.

Assumptions:
- *Sphericity:* The variances of the differences between all combinations of related groups (levels) are equal.
- *Normality:* The dependent variable should be approximately normally distributed within each level of the within-subjects factor.
- *Independence:* Observations are independent of each other.

Steps to perform repeated measures ANOVA:
1. *Formulate hypotheses:* Define the null and alternative hypotheses.
2. *Calculate ANOVA:*
   - *Sum of squares:* Calculate the SS for the within-subjects factor, the error, and the total.
   - *Degrees of freedom (df):* Determine the degrees of freedom for each source of variation.

- *Mean squares:* Calculate the MS by dividing the SS by the corresponding degrees of freedom.
- *F-statistic:* Compute the F-statistic for the within-subjects factor.
3. *Compare F-statistic:* Compare the calculated F-statistic to the critical value from the F-distribution table.
4. *Interpretation:* Determine if the within-subjects factor has a significant effect on the dependent variable.

Illustration:
Comparing IOP before exercise, 1 hour after exercise, and 3 hours after exercise.

TABLE 10.7(a): Table depicting repeated measures ANOVA test applied for the UCVA preoperative and postoperative and group-to-group comparisons was done by post-hoc test (Bonferroni).

UCVA over time preoperative and postoperative.		
Time	UCVA	p-value for repeated measures
Preoperative: Mean ± SD	1.1 ± 0.34	<0.0001
Postoperative 1 month: Mean ± SD	1.02 ± 0.21	
Postoperative 3 month: Mean ± SD	0.86 ± 0.08	
Postoperative 6 month: Mean ± SD	0.82 ± 0.11	
Postoperative 12 month: Mean ± SD	0.72 ± 0.15	
P1 = 0.003, P2 < 0.0001, P3<0.0001, P4 = 0.006, P5 < 0.0001, P6 < 0.0001		
Note: P1: compared preoperative and postoperative 3 month, P2: compared preoperative and postoperative 6 month, P3: compared preoperative and postoperative 12 month, P4: compared postoperative 3 month and postoperative 6 month, P5: compared postoperative 3 month and postoperative 12 month, P6: compared postoperative 6 month and postoperative 12 month (ANOVA: analysis of variance; UCVA: uncorrected visual acuity)		

■ NONPARAMETRIC TESTS

Nonparametric tests are essential tools in the field of ophthalmology, especially when dealing with small sample sizes, ordinal data, or data that do not follow a normal distribution. These tests do not rely on parameter estimates that assume a specific distribution, making them versatile and robust for various types of data. They are particularly useful in clinical studies where assumptions of normality are often violated **(Flowchart 10.1)**.

One common nonparametric test used in ophthalmology is the Mann-Whitney U test. This test is advantageous when comparing two independent groups to discern if there is a significant difference between them, without assuming normal distribution of the data. For instance, in studies comparing the effectiveness of different treatments on visual acuity, nonparametric tests can provide meaningful insights despite the variability and complexity of the data.

TABLE 10.7(b): Explaining **Table 10.7a:** Table depicting repeated measures ANOVA test applied for the UCVA preoperative and postoperative and group-to-group comparisons was done by post-hoc test (Bonferroni).

Clinical outcomes of combined simultaneous femtosecond Kerarings implantation and corneal collagen cross-linking in advanced keratoconus:	
Importance of repeated measures ANOVA	• Repeated measures ANOVA is crucial for analyzing data where the same subjects are tested multiple times. It reduces error variance by using the same subjects across conditions, providing a more powerful test • In the above example comparing improvement in UCVA pre- and postoperative simultaneous femtosecond Kerarings implantation and corneal collagen cross-linking in advanced keratoconus • As UCVA was repeatedly measured postoperatively 1, 3, 6, and 12 months so RMANOVA has been applied and improvement in UCVA is significant
(ANOVA: analysis of variance; RMANOVA: repeated measures ANOVA; UCVA: uncorrected visual acuity)	

Mann-Whitney U Test

The Mann-Whitney U test, also known as the Wilcoxon rank-sum test, is a nonparametric test used to determine whether there is a significant difference between the distributions of two independent groups. Unlike parametric tests, it does not assume that the data follows a normal distribution. Instead, it compares the ranks of values in the two groups. This test is particularly useful when the sample sizes are small, or when the data is ordinal or not normally distributed. The test calculates the U statistic, which is then compared to a critical value from the Mann-Whitney U distribution to determine the p-value. A low p-value indicates that the null hypothesis, which states that the distributions of the two groups are equal, can be rejected.

To perform the Mann-Whitney U test for ophthalmology data, follow these steps:
1. *Collect your data:* Gather the data for two independent groups. For example, suppose we have a study comparing the visual acuity scores of two groups of patients—one treated with aflibercept and the other with ranibizumab **(Tables 10.8a and 10.8b)**.
2. *Rank the data:* Combine the visual acuity scores of both groups and rank them in ascending order. Assign ranks from 1 to N (where N is the total number of observations). If there are tied ranks, assign the average rank to each tied score.
3. *Sum the ranks:* Calculate the sum of the ranks for each group. Let R1 be the sum of the ranks for the aflibercept group and R2 be the sum of the ranks for the ranibizumab group.

4. *Calculate the U statistic:* Use the following formulas to calculate the U statistics for each group:

$$U_1 = n_1 \times n_2 + (n_1 \times (n_1 + 1))/2 - R_1$$
$$U_2 = n_1 \times n_2 - U_1$$

Here, n_1 and n_2 are the sample sizes of the two groups.

5. *Determine the smaller U value:* The Mann-Whitney U statistic is the smaller value between U1 and U2.
6. *Compare to critical value:* Compare the U statistic to the critical value from the Mann-Whitney U distribution table based on the sample sizes and chosen significance level (e.g., 0.05).
7. *Interpret the p-value:* If the U statistic is smaller than the critical value, reject the null hypothesis, indicating a significant difference between the distributions of the two groups.

TABLE 10.8a: Illustration of application of Mann-Whitney U test for retinitis pigmentosa and controls.

Characteristics of retinitis pigmentosa patients with and without optic disc drusen and controls					
	Retinitis pigmentosa			**Controls**	**p-value**
Patients, n (% male)	32 (59)			13 (39)	
Age, years	47 ± 16			49 ± 12	0.802[a]
Macular RNFL, μm	66.9 ± 16.2			38.4 ± 5.2	<0.001[b]
	With ODD		Without ODD		
Patients, n (% male)	12 (50)		18 (61)		
Age, years	40 (38–57)		54 (43–61)		0.175[a]
Goldmann VF, cm²	5.1 (3.4–33.6)		8.4 (1.0–31.9)		0.440[c]
Macular RNFL, μm	69.2 (61.1–79.1)		53.5 (43.0–68.0)		0.011[a]
Note: [a]Students t-test, [b]Welch t-test, [c]Mann-Whitney U test (VF: visual field; RNFL: retinal nerve fiber layer; ODD: optic disc drusen)					

TABLE 10.8(b): Explanation to illustrtion in **Table 10.8(a)** representing Mann-Whitney U test for retinitis pigmentosa and controls

This table is published for a study on macular retinal nerve fiber layer thickness in retinitis pigmentosa patients with and without optic disc drusen	
Importance of Mann-Whitney U test	• In the above example, Mann-Whitney U test is used to compare Goldmann visual fields as an indicator of severity of retinitis pigmentosa in patients with and without optic disc drusen • As severity of a disease is a nonparametric qualitative variable, so Mann-Whitney U test was applied

Wilcoxon Signed Rank Test

The Wilcoxon signed rank test is a nonparametric statistical test used to compare two related samples or repeated measurements on a single sample. It evaluates whether their population mean ranks differ. This test is often used when the assumptions of the paired t-test are not met, particularly when the data cannot be assumed to be normally distributed **(Tables 10.9a and 10.9b)**.

The test calculates the differences between paired observations, ranks these differences, and then evaluates whether the ranks of the positive and negative differences are significantly different.

TABLE 10.9A: Illustration of appliication of t-test in a study comparing temporal AOD and nasal AOD (Rifada et al., 2025/02/26).

Comparison of temporal AOD, nasal AOD, and its mean values before and 1-week after LPI procedure				
	Group			
	Pre-LPI (mean ± SD)	1-week post-LPI (mean ± SD)	T-value/Z-score	
Variable	N = 22	N = 22	Wilcoxon	p-value
Temporal AOD500[a]	0.12 ± 0.074	0.22 ± 0.111	5,724	0.0001**
Temporal AOD750[a]	0.20 ± 0.118	0.31 ± 0.143	4,328	0.0001**
Nasal AOD500[b]	0.12 ± 0.070	0.22 ± 0.097	4,112	0.0001**
Nasal AOD750[a]	0.20 ± 0.100	0.32 ± 0.144	5,235	0.0001**
Mean AOD500[b]	0.12 ± 0.066	0.22 ± 0.091	4,015	0.0001**
Mean AOD750[a]	0.20 ± 0.096	0.31 ± 0.144	6,349	0.0001**
Note: [a]Data with normal distribution; [b]data with abnormal distribution. The temporal AOD500, temporal AOD750, nasal AOD750, and mean AOD750 variables were tested using a paired t-test. The nasal AOD500 and mean AOD500 variables were tested using Wilcoxon alternative test. It was considered significant if p-value < 0.05. *means the result is statistically significant for significance <0.05, **for significance <0.01. (AOD: angle opening distance)				

TABLE 10.9(b): Explaining **Table 10.9(a)**: Comparison of temporal AOD and nasal AOD by using t-test.

In a study on glaucoma evaluating the effectiveness of laser peripheral iridotomy on angle-closure diseases: The role of spectral domain anterior segment optical coherence tomography (SD AS-OCT)	
Choice of Wilcoxon versus t-test	As mentioned in the superscript "b" in < variable [b] > data which are not normally distributed are tested by Wilcoxon signed rank test
(AOD: angle opening distance)	

The Wilcoxon signed rank test involves the following steps:
1. Calculate the differences between each pair of observations.
2. Rank the absolute differences from smallest to largest, ignoring the signs.
3. Assign signs to the ranks based on the original differences' signs.
4. Sum the positive ranks and the negative ranks.
5. Calculate the test statistic (W), which is the smaller of the absolute values of the sums of the positive and negative ranks.
6. Compare the test statistic to the critical value from the Wilcoxon signed rank test table based on the sample size (n) and the chosen significance level (α, typically 0.05).

If the test statistic is less than or equal to the critical value, the null hypothesis (that there is no difference in the median of the paired differences) is rejected.

Mood's Median Test

Mood's median test is a nonparametric statistical test used to determine if there are differences in the medians among two or more independent groups. Unlike other tests that assume normal distributions, Mood's median test is particularly useful when dealing with skewed data or when the sample sizes are small. The test involves calculating the overall median of all observations and then counting how many observations in each group fall above and below this median. These counts are then analyzed using a Chi-squared test to check for significant differences in the medians across the groups. This makes Mood's median test a robust alternative when the assumptions of parametric tests are not met **(Table 10.10)**.

TABLE 10.10: Steps to perform Mood's median test for ophthalmology data, follow these steps.

Step	Description
1. Collect data	Gather your independent groups' data, ensuring they represent different treatments or conditions in ophthalmology
2. Calculate overall median	Compute the median of all observations combined, regardless of their group affiliation
3. Count observations	For each group, count how many observations are above and below the overall median
4. Construct contingency table	Create a table with the counts from each group above and below the median
5. Apply Chi-squared test	Use a Chi-squared test to analyze the contingency table and determine if there are significant differences in the medians across the groups
6. Interpret results	Compare the Chi-squared test statistic to the critical value to decide if the null hypothesis can be rejected

Kruskal–Wallis H Test

The Kruskal–Wallis H test is a rank-based nonparametric test used to determine if there are statistically significant differences between the medians of three or more independent groups. It serves as an extension of the Mann-Whitney U test and is particularly useful when the assumptions for ANOVA (analysis of variance) cannot be met, such as when the data is not normally distributed or when the sample sizes are small and unequal **(Tables 10.11a and 10.11b)**.

To perform the Kruskal–Wallis H Test, all the data points from all groups are ranked together. The test then compares the sum of these ranks across the groups. Specifically, the test evaluates whether the distribution of ranks differs significantly between the groups.

A significant result from the Kruskal–Wallis H Test indicates that at least one group median is different from the others, but it does not specify which groups are different. To pinpoint the specific differences, post-hoc tests can be conducted.

TABLE 10.11(a): Kruskal–Wallis H test (A. et al., 2024/06/01).

	RNFL thickness measurements based on axial length (AL) groups			
	Axial length (AL) groups			
Measurements	**AL<21** 8	**AL 21–24** 31	**AL >24** 30	**p-value**
RNFL average thickness: Mean ±SD	109 ± 9.2	102.6 ± 6	96 ± 6.7	<0.0001**
Post hoc tests	p1 = 0.04, p2 < 0.001, p3 = 0.001			
RNFL superior quadrant: Mean ±SD	137.4 ± 16	127 ± 11.3	111.5 ± 14	<0.0001**
Post hoc tests	p1 = 0.12, p2 < 0.001, p3 < 0.001			
RNFL inferior quadrant: Mean ±SD	136.3 ± 18	126 ± 10.6	119.2 ± 13	0.003*
Post hoc tests	p1 = 0.11, p2 = 0.004, p3 = 0.11			
RNFL nasal quadrant: Mean ±SD	84.9 ± 19	81.4 ± 7.9	75.6 ± 14.8	0.099
Post hoc tests	p1 = 0.77, p2 = 0.17, p3 = 0.2			
RNFL temporal quadrant: Mean ±SD Median (range)	83.4 ± 15.8 81.5 (61–113)	75.6 ± 7 74 (62–92)	79 ± 18 75 (58–154)	0.28
Post hoc tests	p1–0.34, p2–0.73, p3–0.57			
p1 = AL<21 vs. AL 21–24; p2 = AL<21 vs. AL >24; p3 = AL21–24 vs. AL>24 (RNFL: retinal nerve fiber layer) *means the result is statistically significant for significance <0.05, **for significance <0.01.				

TABLE 10.11(b): Explanation to **Table 10.11(a)** for application of Kruskal–Wallis H test (A. et al., 2024/06/01).

In a study comparing effect of axial length on peripapillary retinal nerve fiber layer (RNFL) using optical coherence tomography (OCT)	
Importance of Kruskal–Wallis test	• It is a nonparametric test similar to a one-way ANOVA but for data that is not normally distributed. It can be applied when there are three groups and one variable included, to test for significance • In the illustration above, the Kruskal–Wallis H Test has been applied to the dataset to determine the effect of axial length on RNFL thickness
(ANOVA: analysis of variance)	

Given its nonparametric nature, the Kruskal–Wallis H Test is suitable for ordinal data or data that do not meet the parametric assumptions of ANOVA, making it a versatile tool in statistical analysis.

Difference between Kruskal–Wallis H Test and Mood's Median Test

Kruskal–Wallis H test and Mood's median test are both nonparametric tests used to compare more than two groups, but they differ in their approach and assumptions. The Kruskal–Wallis H test is an extension of the Mann-Whitney U test and is used to determine if there are statistically significant differences between the medians of three or more independent groups. It ranks all the data points from all groups together and then compares the sum of ranks between groups.

On the other hand, Mood's median test is also used to compare the medians of multiple groups, but it evaluates whether the medians are significantly different by comparing how many observations in each group fall above or below the overall median. This test is less sensitive to outliers than the Kruskal–Wallis H test **(Table 10.12)**.

TABLE 10.12: Differentiation between Kruskal–Wallis H test and Mood's median test.

Test	Type	Purpose	Method	Sensitivity	Assumptions
Kruskal–Wallis H test	Nonparametric	Compare medians of 3+ groups	Ranks data points, compares sum of ranks	More sensitive to outliers	No normal distribution assumption
Mood's median test	Nonparametric	Compare medians of multiple groups	Compares observations above/below median	Less sensitive to outliers	No normal distribution assumption

Both tests do not assume a normal distribution of the data, making them suitable for ordinal data or data that do not meet parametric assumptions.

Friedman Test

The Friedman test is a nonparametric alternative to the *one-way ANOVA with repeated measures*. It is used to detect differences in treatments across multiple test attempts. Unlike the Kruskal–Wallis H test, which evaluates differences between groups, the Friedman test focuses on differences within subjects. It is particularly useful when the assumptions for repeated measures ANOVA cannot be met, such as when the data are not normally distributed.

To perform the Friedman test, rankings of each treatment are assigned within each block (or subject), and the test evaluates whether the sum of the ranks differs significantly across treatments. A significant result indicates that at least one treatment is different, but does not specify which treatments are different, requiring post-hoc tests to determine specific differences **[Tables 10.13(a) and 10.13(b)]**.

TABLE 10.13(a): Table showing Friedman (one-way ANOVA) test comparing changes in multiple parameters like macular retinal thickness, choroidal subfoveal thickness, and change in FAZ area, in patients post COVID-19 infection.

Dynamics of retinal and choroidal morphological and morphometric changes in post-COVID-19 patients				
Characteristic	1 month after recovery (n = 104)	6 months after recovery (n = 104)	12 months after recovery (n = 104)	p-value
Macular retinal thickness, μm	252.65 (248.3–257.6)	243.8 (241.15–246.6)	236.25 (232.2–238.55)	<0.001
Choroidal subfoveal thickness, μm	385.25 (381.35–391.25)	346.95 (339.5–354.6)	316.55 (309.5–325.9)	<0.001
FAZ area, mm^2	0.35 (0.295–0.41)	0.44 (0.39–0.51)	0.525 (0.44–0.59)	<0.001
SCP vessel density (6×6 mm scan), %	14.75 (8.6–21.75)	20.45 (13.8–26.4)	25.95 (19.45–33.55)	<0.001
DCP vessel density (6×6 mm scan), %	9.7 (6.3–12.8)	13.75 (10.15–16.85)	17.9 (14.65–21.4)	<0.001
(ANOVA: analysis of variance; DCP: deep capillary plexus; FAZ: foveal avascular zone; SCP: superficial capillary plexus)				

TABLE 10.13b: Explanation to **Table 10.13a**: Table showing Friedman (one-way ANOVA) test comparing changes in multiple parameters like macular retinal thickness, choroidal subfoveal thickness, and change in FAZ area, in patients post COVID-19 infection.

In a study showing "dynamics and features of retinal and choroidal morphological and morphometric changes in post-COVID-19 patients with different variants of the angiotensin-converting enzyme gene"	
Importance of Friedman (one-way ANOVA)	Friedman one-way ANOVA is used to analyze differences within subjects across multiple test attempts without assuming the data's normal distribution. This is particularly crucial in medical research where repeated measures on the same subjects are common, such as in the study of retinal and choroidal changes in post-COVID-19 patients. The Friedman test provides detailed statistical analysis in various retinal and choroidal parameters over a period of time
(ANOVA: analysis of variance)	

Fisher Exact T-test

The Fisher exact test is a statistical significance test used to determine if there are nonrandom associations between two categorical variables. Unlike other tests that require larger sample sizes to validate the results through approximation, the Fisher exact test is particularly useful for small sample sizes and when the data falls into a 2 × 2 contingency table.

This test calculates the exact probability of obtaining a distribution of values in the contingency table more extreme or as extreme as the observed distribution, given the null hypothesis of no association between the variables. The Fisher exact test is an alternative to the Chi-square test when the sample size is small and the expected frequencies in any of the cells of the contingency table are less than 5 **[Tables 10.14(a) and 10.14(b)]**.

One of the key advantages of the Fisher exact test is its accuracy with small sample sizes, making it a robust choice for analyzing categorical data in various fields such as medicine, biology, and social sciences. However, it is computationally intensive, especially for larger tables, and is typically reserved for 2 × 2 tables where other less computational methods may not be suitable.

STATISTICAL SIGNIFICANCE VERSUS CLINICAL SIGNIFICANCE

While the *p*-value and statistical significance play a crucial role in determining whether a study's findings are likely due to chance, they do not necessarily imply practical or clinical importance. Statistical significance indicates that there is a measurable effect or difference, often assessed by a *p*-value

TABLE 10.14(a): Illustration of application of Fisher exact test

Comparison of baseline demographic and clinical characteristics between the two groups			
Variable	Group 1 (mean ± SD) n (%)	Group 2 (mean ± SD) n (%)	p-value
Age	56.08 ± 9.84	53.32 ± 14.13	0.73*
Sex — Male	13 (52%)	15 (60%)	
Sex — Female	12 (48%)	10 (40%)	0.78^
Sex — Total	25 (100%)	25 (100%)	
IOP (mm Hg)	28.40 ± 3.46	28.00 ± 4.30	0.46**
BCVA (LogMAR)	0.5 ± 0.3	0.6 ± 0.2	0.94*
Number of medications	1.88 ± 1.05	1.80 ± 1.12	0.84*

Note: *Mann-Whitney U-test was used, **Kruskal–Wallis one way ANNOVA test was used, ^Fisher exact test was used
(ANOVA: analysis of variance; BCVA: best-corrected visual acuity; IOP: intraocular pressure; LogMAR: logarithm of the minimum angle of resolution)

TABLE 10.14(b): Explanation to **Table 10.14(a):** Table showing Friedman (one-way ANOVA) test comparing changes in multiple parameters like macular retinal thickness, choroidal subfoveal thickness, and change in FAZ area, in patients post COVID-19 infection.

In a study comparing IOP control in primary open angle glaucoma patients undergoing Ex-PRESS mini shunt implantation and deep sclerotomy	
Importance of Fisher exact test	• In the above illustration, Fisher exact test has been applied to test if any statistically significant difference exists between the sex distribution in group A and B patients. The result was in significant • Fisher exact test is used as sex is a qualitative data not normally distributed

(ANOVA: analysis of variance; FAZ: foveal avascular zone)

threshold such as 0.05. However, this does not always translate to clinical significance, which refers to the actual relevance or impact of the findings on patient care and outcomes.

For example, a study might find a statistically significant difference in IOP reduction between two treatments for glaucoma, with a p-value of 0.03. However, if the reduction in IOP is minimal and does not lead to a substantial improvement in patients' vision or quality of life, the clinical significance is limited. Therefore, ophthalmologists must consider both statistical and clinical significance when evaluating new treatments or interventions.

Clinical significance often involves the magnitude of the effect, the practical implications for daily medical practice, and whether the findings translate into meaningful health benefits for patients. It is possible to have statistically significant results with negligible clinical impact, or vice versa, where a treatment shows a large and beneficial effect that may not meet the strict criteria for statistical significance due to sample size or study design limitations.

Ultimately, balancing statistical rigor with clinical relevance ensures that research findings are both scientifically valid and practically beneficial for patient care in ophthalmology, guiding informed decision-making and improving outcomes.

Is a statistically significant 1 mm Hg difference of IOP shown to be 10% beneficial always to be considered as clinically significant?

In the context of lowering IOP in glaucoma patients, a reduction of 1 mm Hg can be evaluated from both statistical and clinical significance perspectives. Statistically, if the *p*-value associated with this reduction is below a predetermined threshold, such as 0.05, the result is considered statistically significant, meaning that the observed effect is unlikely to be due to chance.

However, the clinical significance of a 1 mm Hg reduction is crucial to consider. Clinically, ophthalmologists assess whether this reduction translates into meaningful health benefits for the patient, such as improved vision, decreased risk of glaucoma progression, or enhanced quality of life. A 1 mm Hg decrease may be deemed clinically significant if it contributes to a substantial improvement in the patient's condition or if it adds to the cumulative effect of other treatments in managing glaucoma effectively **(Table 10.15)**.

TABLE 10.15: Steps in diagnostic test performance metrics for analyzing diagnostic reliability through sensitivity and specificity.

Step	Description
Collect data	Gather results of diagnostic test, including TP, FP, TN, FN
Calculate sensitivity	Sensitivity = TP/(TP + FN)
Calculate specificity	Specificity = TN/(TN + FP)
Determine *p*-values	Use statistical tests (e.g., Chi-square) to calculate *p*-values for sensitivity and specificity
Calculate confidence intervals	Use the formula for the confidence interval of a proportion
Interpret results	Analyze *p*-values and confidence intervals to understand reliability and precision

(FN: false negatives; FP: false positives; TN: true negatives; TP: true positives)

■ INTERPRETING ACCURACY OF DIAGNOSTIC TESTS

To calculate sensitivity, specificity, *p*-values, and confidence intervals, you can follow these steps:

1. *Collect data:* Gather the results of your diagnostic test, including true positives (TP), false positives (FP), true negatives (TN), and false negatives (FN).
2. *Calculate sensitivity and specificity:*
   - *Sensitivity:* Sensitivity = $\dfrac{TP}{TP + FN}$
   - *Specificity:* Specificity = $\dfrac{TN}{TN + FP}$
3. *Determine p-values:* Use statistical tests (e.g., Chi-square test) to calculate the *p*-values for sensitivity and specificity. This helps determine if the observed values are statistically significant.
4. *Calculate confidence intervals:*
   - *For sensitivity:* Use the formula for the confidence interval of a proportion.
   - *For specificity:* Similarly, use the formula for the confidence interval of a proportion.

   The formula for a 95% confidence interval for a proportion p is: CI = p ± Zp (1 – p) where Z is the Z-score corresponding to the desired confidence level (e.g., 1.96 for 95%), and n is the sample size.
5. *Interpret results:* Analyze the *p*-values and confidence intervals to understand the reliability and precision of your sensitivity and specificity estimates.

■ OVERVIEW OF TESTS TO BE APPLIED PARAMETRIC AND NONPARAMETRIC

The tests that the statisticians usually apply for parametric and nonparametric tests are based on several factors and algorithmically summarized in **Flowchart 10.1**.

Tests of normality also have a crucial role to play in the algorithm.

- If SD is < half of mean, then data is normally distributed. Test with Sapiro wilk if N <2,000 or Kolmogorov Smirnov test if N >2,000. Tests for correlation (degrees of relationship): Normally distributed use Spearman's rank correlation.
- For data which is not normally distributed use Spearman's rank correlation. For statistically significant results, you can further analyze using multilinear or multinomial regression, if the data is normally

Flowchart 10.1: Classification of the tests (parametric and nonparametric) based on the data type.

distributed. If not, convert the data into log values and then perform regression.

CONCLUSION

In summary, the application of both parametric and nonparametric tests, guided by tests of normality and correlation, provides robust tools for statistical analysis. The careful selection and interpretation of these tests ensure the reliability and precision of the results. As we delve deeper into understanding complex data, the importance of these statistical methods becomes paramount, guiding us toward more accurate and meaningful conclusions.

BIBLIOGRAPHY

1. Abdelwhad N, Mohamed M, Yousef H, Mounir A. Clinical outcomes of combined simultaneous femtosecond kerarings implantation and corneal collagen cross-linking in advanced keratoconus. Egypt J Clin Ophthalmol [Internet]. 2021 (cited 2021/12/01);4(2). Available from: https://doi.org/10.21608/ejco.2021.215518
2. Hutsaliuk KM, Rossokha ZI, Skalska NI, Ulianova NA. Dynamics and features of retinal and choroidal morphological and morphometric changes in post-COVID-19 patients with different variants of the angiotensin-converting enzyme gene. Oftalmologicheskii Zhurnal [Internet]. 2025 (cited 2025);114(1):9-16. Available from: https://doi.org/10.31288/oftalmolzh20251916
3. Joshi M, Naik MP, Sarkar L. Effect of intravitreal anti-vascular endothelial growth factor on corneal endothelial cell count and central corneal thickness in Indian population. J Family Med Prim Care [Internet]. 2019 (cited 2019);8(7):2429-32. Available from: https://doi.org/10.4103/jfmpc.jfmpc_314_19
4. Khallaf H, Abdel Badie M, El-moddather M, Gad El kareem A. Comparison between ex-press mini shunt implantation and deep sclerotomy in patients with primary open-angle glaucoma (POAG). Egypt J Clin Ophthalmol [Internet]. 2021 (cited 2021/12/01);4(2):57-65. Available from: https://doi.org/10.21608/ejco.2021.215520
5. Mustafa A, Mostafa E, Mounir A, Mostafa A. Effect of axial length on pripapillary retinal nerve fibre layer (RNFL) using optical coherence tomography (OCT). Egypt J Clin Ophthalmol [Internet]. 2024 (cited 2024/06/01);7(1). Available from: https://doi.org/10.21608/ejco.2024.361188
6. Rifada M, Ramdhani RF, Nadifa I, Gustianty E, Umbara S, Prahasta A, et al. Evaluating the Effectiveness of Laser Peripheral Iridotomy on Angle-closure Diseases: The Role of Spectral Domain Anterior Segment Optical Coherence Tomography (SD AS-OCT) in Indonesia Tertiary Eye Hospital. Open Ophthalmol J [Internet]. 2025 (cited 2025/02/26);19(1). Available from: https://doi.org/10.2174/0118743641337429241016053642
7. Steensberg AH, Malmqvist L, Bertelsen M, Kessel L, Grønskov K, Hamann S. Frontiers | Macular retinal nerve fiber layer thickness in retinitis pigmentosa patients with and without optic disc drusen. Front Ophthalmol [Internet].

2024 (cited 2024/12/05);4. Available from: https://doi.org/10.3389/fopht.2024.1476911

8. Ye Y, Hu Z, Su N, Shen Y, Yuan S. Frontiers | Axial length to corneal curvature radius ratio is negatively correlated with choroidal blood flow in myopic children. Front Ophthalmol [Internet]. 2025 (cited 2025/01/06);4. Available from: https://doi.org/10.3389/fopht.2024.1540410

9. Zimmermann CM, Cardakli N, Kraus CL. Frontiers | Cup-to-disc ratio measured clinically and via OCT in pediatric patients being monitored as glaucoma suspects for suspicious optic discs. Front Ophthalmol [Internet]. 2024 (cited 2024/12/03);4. Available from: https://doi.org/10.3389/fopht.2024.1479286

CHAPTER 11

Sample Size Determination

Ajay Sharma, Durga Bhavani Mummina

■ INTRODUCTION

As an ophthalmologist, understanding the intricacies of clinical research is pivotal to advancing patient care and contributing to the broader medical community. One of the fundamental aspects of designing a robust clinical study is determining the appropriate sample size, which ensures the validity and reliability of the study's outcomes. Proper sample size calculation can influence the credibility of findings, the ethical use of resources, and the overall impact of the research. This chapter delves into the critical elements of sample size determination, providing a comprehensive guide that underscores its importance in the context of ophthalmologic studies.

Moreover, sample size determination is essential for ensuring ethical standards in research. By calculating the right sample size, researchers can avoid the pitfalls of underpowered studies that may lead to inconclusive results or overpowered studies that waste resources. It also helps in minimizing the risk of type I and type II errors, enhancing the study's precision and accuracy.

In the realm of ophthalmology, where patient outcomes can be significantly influenced by clinical decisions, the importance of precise and reliable data cannot be overstated. Whether investigating the efficacy of a new glaucoma treatment or assessing the impact of a surgical procedure on visual acuity, the accuracy of your findings hinges on the robustness of your sample size calculations. This chapter will explore the basic concepts and provide practical examples to aid in the design of effective and impactful ophthalmologic research.

■ BASIC CONCEPTS FOR SAMPLE SIZE CALCULATIONS

Expected Difference (d)

The *Expected Difference (d)*, also known as the *effect size*, is a key parameter in sample size calculations. It represents the magnitude of the difference you expect to detect between groups or conditions in your study. This could be the difference in means, proportions, or other measures of interest.

For example, if you compare the average intraocular pressure (IOP) between two groups, the expected difference would be the difference in average IOP you anticipate observing. The larger the expected difference, the smaller the sample size needed to detect it, and vice versa.

Variability (S_d)

Variability refers to how spread out or dispersed the data points are in a dataset. In the context of sample size calculation, it is a measure of the extent to which individual observations in a sample differ from the sample mean. High variability means that the data points are spread out over a wide range of values, while low variability indicates that the data points are clustered closely around the mean.

Type I Error/Level of Significance

- *Type I error (α)*: This is the probability of rejecting the null hypothesis when it is actually true. It represents the likelihood of a false positive. A common choice for α is 0.05, which means there is a 5% risk of concluding that there is an effect when there is none.
- *Level of significance ($Z_{1-\alpha/2}$)*: This value corresponds to the critical value of the standard normal distribution for a given α. For example, if α is 0.05, then $Z_{1-\alpha/2}$ is approximately 1.96. This critical value is used to determine the margin of error and the confidence interval **(Table 11.1)**.

Type II Error/Power ($Z_{1-\beta}$)

- *Type II error*: A type II error occurs when the test fails to reject a false null hypothesis (i.e., it misses an effect that is actually there). The probability of a type II error is denoted by β. Minimizing β is important, because it increases the reliability of the test results. A high β means a higher chance of missing a true effect, which can lead to incorrect conclusions **(Table 11.2)**.
- *Power of the test:* The power of a test is the probability that it correctly rejects a false null hypothesis (i.e., it detects an effect when there is one). High power reduces the risk of a type II error. It ensures that the study is sensitive enough to detect meaningful differences or effects. A typical target for power is 80% or higher, meaning there is an 80% chance of detecting an effect if it exists **(Table 11.3)**.
- *Note:* Power is calculated as $1-\beta$. Therefore, as the power of the test increases, the probability of a type II error decreases.

Z-values (or) Standard Normal Table Values for Level of Significance (α) and Power ($1 - \beta$)

TABLE 11.1: Contingency table (2*2).

		True state of nature (when it is true)	
		H_0	H_a
Acceptance/ conclusion	H_0	Accept (True positive)	Type II error (False negative)
	H_a	Type I error (False positive)	Accept (True negative)

Sample Size Determination

TABLE 11.2: Standard normal table values with respect to level of significance (LoS).

LoS	Z values for specific LoS	
	Two tailed	One tailed
0.05	1.96	1.65
0.01	2.58	2.33

TABLE 11.3: Standard normal table values with respect to power.

Power (1-β) [in %]	β	$Z_{1-\beta}$ values
80	0.2	0.84
90	0.1	1.28
95	0.05	1.64

SAMPLE SIZE COMPUTATION FOR INDEPENDENT SAMPLE T-TEST

When the two Groups are Independent

$$n = \frac{2\left[(Z_{1-\frac{\alpha}{2}}) + (Z_{1-\beta})\right]^2}{\left(\dfrac{d}{s}\right)^2}$$

There are situations in which the reteach group wants *unequal number in each group* say in 1:k ratio, i.e., $n_2 = k\,n_1$. Then the sample size n_1 for group 1 is estimated using the formula **Tables 11.4(a) and 11.4 (b)**.

TABLE 11.4a: Illustration of sample size calculation needs in two independent groups (Li et al., 2025/01/01).

	Baseline demographic data of completed subjects			
	DIMS (n = 72)	SV (n = 79)	p value	Effect size
Age (years)	10.69 (10.33~11.06)	10.38 (10.00~10.76)	0.237	−0.19 (−0.51~0.13)
Gender, male/female	43/30	44/35	0.744	—
SER (D)	−3.16 (−3.54~−2.78)	−3.13 (−3.49~−2.77)	0.910	0.02 (−0.30~0.34)
Axial length (mm)	24.82 (24.62~25.03)	25.02 (24.79~25.26)	0.204	0.21 (−0.11~0.53)
Flat keratometry (D)	42.66 (42.30~43.02)	42.64 (42.33~42.95)	0.925	−0.02 (−0.34~0.30)
Steep keratometry (D)	43.98 (43.60~44.36)	43.85 (43.50~44.20)	0.617	−0.08 (−0.40~0.24)
Total QIRC score	54.29 (52.31~56.28)	51.84 (49.82~53.85)	0.087	−0.28 (−0.60~0.04)

Note: The data are represented by mean (95% CI). All variables were analyzed by unpaired t-test except for gender, which was analyzed by χ^2 test. The effect sizes were represented as Cohen's *d*, the same follow as.
(D: diopters: DIMS: defocus incorporated multiple segments lens: QIRC: Quality of Life Impact of Refractive Correction; SER: spherical equivalent refraction; SV: single vision lens)
Source: Muijzer MB, et al.

TABLE 11.4(b): Explaining, the illustration of sample size calculation needs in two independent groups.

Sample size calculation in situations where two groups are independent and equal/similar in number	A 2-year study noted a 0.50D (SD 0.70D) difference in myopia progression between groups. For 1-year study, we aimed for a medium effect size (Cohen's $d \approx 0.5$) with 62 subjects per group to achieve 80% power and 0.05 significance. To account for a 20% dropout rate, each group required 75 participants.
Source: Li X, et al.	

TABLE 11.5(a): Illustration of sample size calculation needs two independent groups with unequal numbers of subjects.

	Comparison of BCVA among the studied groups					
	Patients group (No. = 50)		Control group (No. = 25)		Independent t test	
	Mean	SD	Mean	SD	t	p value
BCVA	0.21	0.11	0.94	0.05	−31.407	<0.001
Comparison between patients group and control group among CMT, ORL, and SFCT						
	Patients group (No. = 50)		Control group (No. = 25)		Independent t test	
	Mean	SD	Mean	SD	t	p value
CMT (µm)	393.94	72.57	227.36	4.82	11.425	<0.001
ORL (µm)	73.10	9.17	110.56	4.10	−19.434	<0.001
SFCT (µm)	200.68	42.73	249.08	4.64	−5.628	<0.001

(CMT: central macular thickness; ORL: outer retinal layer; SFT: subfoveal choroidal thickness)
Source: Yousef H, et al.

TABLE 11.5b: Illustration of sample size calculation needs two independent groups with unequal numbers of subjects.

	Sample Size Calculation in Situations where two Groups are Independent and *not Equal* in Number

Unequal Number of Samples in two Groups

While discussing unequal number of samples, we can consider the below formula for the independent sample groups. The concept is illusterated **(Tables 11.5a and 11.5b)** from study by (H. et al., 2024/12/01).

$$n = \frac{\left(1+\frac{1}{k}\right)\left[(Z_{1-\frac{\alpha}{2}})+(Z_{1-\beta})\right]^2}{\left(\frac{d}{s}\right)^2}$$

The reason a different formula is applied for sample size calculation when there are unequal numbers in the control and experimental groups is due to the need for adjusting statistical power and precision. When groups are unequal, the balance between the groups changes, which can affect the study's ability to detect a difference between them.

In an equal group scenario, the sample size calculation assumes uniform distribution and equal variances, leading to straightforward power estimation. However, when one group outnumbers the other (in a 1:k ratio), the statistical power and effect size calculations must account for this imbalance to avoid bias and ensure accuracy.

The formula for unequal sample sizes typically includes adjustments that reflect the different group sizes. This ensures that the significance level (α) and the power ($1-\beta$) of the test are maintained appropriately, considering the proportional difference between the groups. This adjustment helps in achieving more precise and reliable results, even when the sample sizes are not equivalent.

In summary, the different formula for unequal sample sizes in control and experimental groups is applied to maintain the integrity and accuracy of the statistical analysis, ensuring that the study's findings are valid despite the imbalance.

Control Group Size in Experimental Research

When is Equal Size Necessary and when is a Smaller Control Group Justifiable?
In experimental research, determining the appropriate size of control groups is crucial for the validity and reliability of study results. The size of control groups can either be equal to or smaller than the experimental groups, depending on various factors and research contexts.

Situations where Equal Control Group Size is Necessary
- *Ensuring statistical power and precision:* In studies where both control and experimental groups must yield high statistical power and precision, an equal number of participants is essential. Equal group sizes simplify the calculation of statistical power and significance levels, thus ensuring accurate and reliable results. For example, in randomized controlled trials (RCTs) for drug efficacy, equal group sizes help to minimize variability and distribute random errors evenly across both groups.
- *Uniform distribution and equal variances:* When the study design requires uniform distribution and equal variances, having equal group sizes is critical. This scenario is common in studies using parametric tests, such as t-tests and analysis of variance (ANOVA), where equal variances are an assumption for valid results.
- *Ethical considerations:* In clinical trials and studies involving human subjects, equal group sizes may be necessary to ensure fairness and ethical treatment of participants. Allocating an equal number of participants to

both control and experimental groups ensures that all individuals have an equal chance of receiving the intervention or treatment.

Situations where a Smaller Control Group can be Justified

- *Resource constraints:* In some cases, researchers may face limitations in terms of resources, funding, or time, making it challenging to recruit a large number of participants. A smaller control group can be justified if it still provides sufficient power for detecting meaningful differences while adhering to resource constraints.
- *Pilot studies:* Pilot studies, which are preliminary investigations conducted to test the feasibility of research designs, often have smaller control groups. These studies aim to gather initial data and refine methodologies rather than achieve definitive results. As such, a smaller control group is typically acceptable.
- *High effect size:* When the expected effect size is large, a smaller control group may be sufficient to detect significant differences between groups. In such cases, researchers can achieve adequate statistical power even with unequal group sizes, as the large effect size compensates for the smaller number of control participants.
- *Ethical and practical considerations:* In certain situations, it may be ethically or practically challenging to recruit a large control group. For instance, in studies involving rare diseases or vulnerable populations, it may not be feasible to have equal group sizes. A smaller control group can be justified if it still allows for meaningful comparisons while addressing ethical and practical concerns.

■ COMPARISON OF TWO DEPENDENT (PAIRED) MEANS

When the two Groups are Dependent

Studies that compare samples based on means before and after interventions are prevalent across various research fields. Examples include comparing conduct scores before and after behavior therapy or assessing happiness levels before and after music therapy sessions. In such studies, the paired t-test is the appropriate analysis method.

Estimating the sample size for paired mean comparisons involves determining the necessary sample size to achieve a specified power level for a given difference between the mean changes under the null hypothesis (H0). This estimation also considers the standard deviation of the change and the significance level (α).

The formula for the sample size n when you compare means of two dependent group is:

$$n = \frac{(Z_{1-\alpha/2} + Z_{1-\beta})^2}{d^2}$$

How to Report the Sample Size Computation?

The sample size for the study was computed using Excel or G*Power. With the expected difference of n units from pre- to post- and standard deviation of ___ units, power 80% and level of significance, sample size for the present study is calculated as ___ subjects (eyes).

Note: Expected difference and standard deviation are individualized for each study. Usually, expected difference and standard deviation are determined from pilot study, or already published literature.

Sample Size for one Way ANOVA

Cohen considered small, medium, and large values of f to be 0.10, 0.25, and 0.40, respectively. According to Cohen, values of f larger as 0.5 is not common behavioral sciences, which need not be true always. The noncentrality parameter $\lambda = f^2 n$ and hence $n = \frac{f^2}{\lambda}$. The sample size for ANOVA is computed based on an iterative procedure. For an initial value of sample size n (say n = 5), and fixed value of effect size f, the value of λ is computed. Once the value of λ is obtained based on the initial value of n, power is computed using noncentral F distribution for fixed level of significance (α). If the computed power is not equal to the required power for the initial value of n, fixed values of f and α, the above procedure will continue for a different value of n. The values of λ and power will be computed. This iteration continues until the computed power is equal to the required power.

In case mean and within standard deviation is σ is not known, one can consider the various levels of effect size defined by Cohen as 0.1 as small effect size, 0.25 as medium effect size and 0.40 as large effect size.

Bonferroni Method of Computing the Sample Size for ANOVA

Bonferroni method is another method of computing sample size for ANOVA by utilizing the sample size formula for independent samples t-test after adjusting for multiple comparisons. This method is called Bonferroni Correction method of estimating sample size **(Tables 11.6a and 11.6b)**.

For example, as there are four groups and six possible comparisons and hence level of significance has to be adjusted for these six comparisons by dividing the α value with the number of comparisons ($ex: \frac{\alpha}{6} = \frac{0.056}{6} = 0.00833$)

The two-sided Z value for the above Bonferroni Corrected α value 2.64

Then the Bonferroni corrected sample size for the $(i, j)^{th}$ group comparison $(i, j = 1, 2, 3, 4, 5, 6, i \neq j)$ is given by:

$$n_{ij} = 2 \left[\frac{(Z_{1-\frac{\alpha}{2r}} + Z_{1-\beta}) S_{ij}}{d_{ij}} \right]^2$$

TABLE 11.6(a): Table depicting 202 sample size for all the three groups was drawn by one-way ANOVA Technique (Ye et al., 2025/01/06).

ANOVA results of the mean axial, AL/CR, and macular fovea choroidal perfusion after grouping by myopia severity		Sum of squares	Degree of freedom	Mean square	F	Significance
Axial* myopia severity	Between Groups	88.802	2	44.401	84.309	0.000
	Intragroup	104.803	199	0.527		
	Total	193.605	201			
AL/CR* myopia severity	Between Groups	1.531	2	0.765	143.555	0.000
	Intragroup	1.061	199	0.005		
	Total	2.591	201			
Macular fovea choroidal perfusion* myopia severity	Between Groups	0.044	2	0.022	10.421	0.000
	Intragroup	0.424	199	0.002		
	Total	0.468	201			
*Represent significance levels of 10% respectively. (AL/CR: Ration of Axial length to corneal curvature radius)						

TABLE 11.6(b): Explanation for the above **Table 11.6(a)**, depicting 202 sample size for all the three groups was drawn by one-way ANOVA Technique (Ye et al., 2025/01/06)

Application of one-way ANOVA methodology to determine the sample size	A total of 202 myopic children aged 6–12 years were included in this study, with only data from the right eye selected for enrollment, resulting in a total of 202 eyes. Among the participants, 85 were boys (42.6% of the total) and 117 were girls (57.4% of the total)
(ANOVA: analysis of variance)	

■ SAMPLE SIZE FOR REPEATED MEASURES ANOVA

The outcome variable is pain score measured using visual analog scale (VAS), which is a continuous variable range from 1 to 100. Hence, the objective is to find whether there is significant change in mean VAS score between the three time points, namely between baseline and 3 months and 6 months. The null hypothesis to be tested is that the mean VAS score is same between the three time points and alternate hypothesis is that the mean VAS score differs between at least any two times points. Paired t test can be used to compare the mean VAS score between baseline and 3 months and between 3 months and 6 months and between baseline and 6 months. But this will inflate the type I error rate as three different paired t-tests are performed for one objective/hypothesis. Hence, we need to use a statistical method called Repeated Measures ANOVA (RMANOVA) to compare the mean pain score between the three time points.

The RMANOVA is an extension of paired t test and is used to compare the mean of a variable measured at two or more time points. The assumptions for RMANOVA are:
- The variable at each time point follows normal distribution.
- *Sphericity assumption:* This assumption requires that the variance of the outcome variable is same at each time points, and also all correlations (ρ) between pairs of repeated measurements are equal.

Testing of Hypothesis

- H_0: The means of the outcome variables are equal between all-time points.
- H_1 or H_a: The means of outcome variable differs between at least two time points.
- *Effect size in RMANOVA:* Effect size can be conceived of as measure of the distance between H_0 and H_1. Hence, effect size refers to the underlying population rather than a specific sample. In specifying an effect size, researchers define the degree of deviation from H_0 that they consider important enough to warrant attention. In other words, effects that are smaller than the specified effect size are considered negligible. The effect size parameter should be specified prior to collecting the data.

The value of effect size to be considered depends on the theoretical context of the research or related research results published previously. Cohen (1998) defines f's of 0.1, 0.25, and 0.4 as small, medium, and large effects, respectively. Moreover, using the published results, the effect size, f, can also be computed from the square root of the ratio of the variance explained by the tested effect to the error variance. Mathematically, f can be defined as:

$$f = \sqrt{\frac{\text{Variance explained by special effect}}{\text{Error variance}}} = \sqrt{\frac{\sigma_k^2}{\sigma^2}} = \frac{\sigma_k}{\sigma}$$

Where $\sigma_k = \sqrt{\frac{\sum_{i=1}^{k}(\mu_i - \bar{\mu})^2}{k}}$, where μ_i denoting the population mean at the ith time point, $\bar{\mu}$ denoting the grand mena or mean of all populations means, and k is the number of time points. The standard deviation, σ of each study population is assumed to be equal. The relation between the standardized effect size measures f or f² to the noncentrality parameter λ of the noncentral F distribution is given by:

$$\lambda = \frac{Nf^2 m}{1-\rho}$$

$$f^2 = \frac{\eta^2}{1-\eta^2}$$

Where is the proportion of variance in the outcome variable that is explained by the special effect (here time) nm and is called the partial eta-squared which is given by:

$$\eta^2 = \frac{\sigma_k^2}{\sigma_k^2 + \sigma^2}$$

Bonferroni Method of Computing the Sample Size for RMANOVA

Another method of computing sample size for RMANOVA is by utilizing the sample size formula for two groups in clinical trials after adjusting for multiple comparisons. This method is called Bonferroni correction method of estimating sample size **(Table 11.7)**.

Let there are only two groups, and the outcome variable is measured at m number of timepoints (for example, m = 3). Then there are τ = m(m - 1)/2 possible comparisons of m time points between the two groups. Let σ^2 is the within-subjects variance at each time point, and d is the anticipated differences between treatment group means at any given time point, and ρ is the correlation among repeated measurements or time points (m). Then the sample size for the (i, j)th comparison is calculated using the following formula.

$$n_{ij} = 2\left[\frac{(Z_{\frac{\alpha}{2\tau}} + Z_\beta)\sigma_{ij}}{d_{ij}}\right]\left[1 + \frac{(m-1)\rho}{m}\right]$$

Where n_{ij}, σ_{ij}, and d_{ij} are respectively the number of subjects required in each of the (i,j)th group, pooled standard deviation of the (i,j)th group, and the minimum clinically significant difference in the (i,j)th group (I,j = 1, 2, 3,...τ, i≠j).

Then the sample size in each group is maximum (n_{ij}).

The above equation is an extension to the sample size formula for comparing mean of two independent groups, with additional terms, including the number of repeated measurements (m) per subject and the variance inflation factor [1+(m-1)ρ], to account for the degree of clustering among observations from the same subject. As ρ increases, the required sample size n increases.

Illustration:

TABLE 11.7: Representation for the RMANOVA.

In a study representing titled "Clinical Outcomes of Combined Simultaneous Femtosecond Kerarings Implantation and Corneal Collagen Cross-linking in Advanced Keratoconus"

This study considered sample size for RMANOVA	This study illustrates that "A total of 25 eyes of 33 patients are subjected to simultaneous combination of accelerated corneal collagen cross-linking and FemtoLASIK Keraring implantation with follow-up for a period of 1 year

■ SAMPLE SIZE FOR ESTIMATING MEAN, PROPORTION

Sample Size for Estimation of Mean

A nutritionist wishes to conduct a survey among a population of teenage girls to determine their average daily protein intake (in grams). The nutritionist would like an internal of 10 g, i.e., the estimate should be within 5 g of the population mean. What sample size is needed if he sets confidence as 95%, and the population standard deviation is about 20 g.

$$N = \left[\frac{Z_{(1-\frac{\alpha}{2})}\sigma}{d}\right]^2$$

Sample Size for Estimation of Proportion

An ophthalmologist wants to conduct a survey with an objective to estimate the prevalence of a particular disease in a population, for example, the prevalence of asthma in young children in a particular locality. An unbiased estimate of the prevalence can be provided if the sample is selected from the population by simple random sampling. In designing such a survey, the epidemiologist is likely to ask: "How many subjects do I need to examine in order to assess prevalence with a reasonable degree of accuracy?".

$$n = \left[\frac{2Z_{1-\alpha\backslash 2}}{d}\right]^2 \times \bar{p}\bar{q}$$

Sample Size for Estimation of Accuracy of Diagnostic Test

Accuracy of a diagnostic test is evaluated by sensitivity and specificity.

Sensitivity is defined as proportion of true positives, i.e., the probability (percentage) that patients with the infection (determined by the result of the reference or: "Gold Standard Test") will have a positive result using the test under evaluation.

Specificity is defined as proportion, sample size for estimating sensitivity alone when the disease status is known, we can use.

$$n = \left[\frac{Z_{1-\alpha/2}}{d}\right]^2 \times \bar{p}\bar{q}$$

Later Buderer incorporated the prevalence-based formula to collect the sufficient sample size.

$$n_{se} = \frac{Z^2_{1-\alpha/2} \times \hat{Se}}{d^2 \times Prevalence}$$

SAMPLE SIZE FOR COMPARISON OF TWO PROPORTIONS: INDEPENDENT AND PAIRED

Equality of two Independent Proportions

Are two competing drugs equally effective?

H_0: (P1 = P2) Proportion of the event under study in population is equal to the proportion of the event under study in other population.

There are various test statistics for testing the above null hypothesis; all these tests follow Z or chi-square distribution.

For Unequal Sample Size

$$n_1 = \frac{\left[Z_{\alpha/2}\sqrt{\bar{p}\bar{q}(1+\frac{1}{k})} + Z_\beta\sqrt{p_1 q_1 + \frac{p_2 q_2}{k}}\right]^2}{\Delta^2}$$

$n_2 = kn_1$
p_1, p_2 = projected true probabilities of success (or proportion of event under study) in the two groups
$q_1 = 1-p_1$ and $q_2 = 1-p_2$
$\Delta = |p_2 - p_1|$ (which is the effect size)

$$\bar{p} = \frac{p1 + kp_2}{1+k}$$

$\bar{q} = 1 - \bar{p}$

For the Equal Sample Size

Consider k = 1 in the above formulae.

Inequality of Proportions between two Dependent Groups (Sample Size for McNemar's Test)

The outcome variable is binary, and study design can be a crossover trial or a matched case–control study or a cross-sectional study in which two groups of individuals are related (husband-wife, sibling, twin studies, etc.)

$$N_{(Pairs)} = \frac{[Z_{\frac{\alpha}{2}}(\varphi+1) + Z_\beta \sqrt{(\phi+1)^2 - (\phi+1)^2 \, II \, Discordant}]^2}{(\phi+1)^2 \, II \, Discordant}$$

SAMPLE SIZE FOR SUPERIORITY, NONINFERIORITY, AND EQUIVALENCE TRIALS

To understand the sample size estimation in the context of superiority, noninferiority, and Equivalence trials **(Table 11.8)**.

TABLE 11.8: Null and alternative hypothesis framing for study designs.

Study type	Null hypotheses (H_0)	Research hypothesis (H_1)
Traditional comparison (of two population means)	There is *no* difference between the therapies $H_0: \mu_A = \mu_B$	There is a difference between the therapies $H_1: \mu_A \neq \mu_B$
Superiority trial	The new therapy is *not* superior to the standard therapy $H_0: \mu_A - \mu_B \leq \delta$	The new therapy is superior to the standard therapy $H_1: \mu_A - \mu_B > \delta$
Noninferiority trial	The new therapy is inferior to the standard therapy $H_0: \mu_A - \mu_B \leq -\delta$	The new therapy is noninferior to the standard therapy $H_1: \mu_A - \mu_B > -\delta$
Equivalence trial: Efficacies of the two therapies are close enough, so that one cannot be considered superior or inferior to the other	The new therapy is *not* equivalent to current therapy $H_0: |\mu_A - \mu_B| > \delta$	The new therapy is equivalent to current therapy $H_1: -\delta < \mu_A - \mu_B < \delta$ $H_1: |\mu_A - \mu_B| \leq \delta$

Randomized Clinical Trials (RCT)

Efficacy of new drugs/treatments is established through RCT.
- A prospective study comparing the effect and value of intervention(s) against a control in human being
- The gold standard for establishing efficacy of a newly developed drug/treatment method

- A well-designed clinical trial should clearly specify type of hypothesis to be tested and procedures to be used for analysis of primary outcomes.
- Specify whether the study is to test the difference between different treatment.

Treatment Conditions

Specify whether the study is to test the difference between different treatment conditions.
- *Superiority (new treatment/intervention is superior to the established intervention):* Detect a significant difference between two treatments.
- *Equivalence (new treatment intervention is equivalent/similar to the established intervention):* Similarity can be quantified using the *tolerance limit range* (mean difference of two treatments is within the tolerance range).
- *Noninferiority (new treatment intervention is no worse than or at least as good as the established intervention):* It shows that the new treatment intervention is not inferior to the established intervention by more than prespecified amount, called the noninferiority margin, or δ.

Sample Size for Superiority or Noninferior: Comparison of two Population Means

$$n = \frac{(k+1)}{k} \frac{\{\sigma^2[Z_{1-\alpha} + Z_{1-\beta}]^2\}}{[|d| - \delta]^2}$$

The quantities $Z_{1-\alpha}$ and $Z_{1-\beta}$ are values from the $N(0, 1)$ corresponding to α and β.
[For $\alpha = 0.05$, $Z_{1-\alpha} = 1.65$ (one-tailed)]
[$Z_{1-\beta}$: Value at specified power ($Z_{0.8} = 0.84$; $Z_{0.9} = 1.28$)]
σ: Pooled standard deviation
d: Anticipated difference in means of the two groups ($\mu_A - \mu_B$)
δ: Margin of clinical significance or testing margin ($\delta < 0$ *for noninferiority and* $\delta > 0$ *for superiority*)
k: Allocation ratio between treatment groups
Note: For a given d, sample sizes increase with higher values of δ.

Sample Size for Superiority or Noninferior: Comparison of two Population Proportions

For comparative studies, it's crucial to define in what context and manner are we examining the effectiveness of different interventions or treatments.

A non-inferiority or superiority. A non-inferiority randomized control trial is illustrated by study from (Muijzer et al., 2023) in **Table 11.9a** to evaluate the use of intraoperative OCT during Descemet membrane endothelial keratoplasty, to study Outcomes of the advanced visualization in corneal surgery. The formulas used are:

TABLE 11.9a: Tabulation for a non-inferiority randomized control trial to evaluate the use of intraoperative OCT during Descemet membrane endothelial keratoplasty, To study Outcomes of the advanced visualization in corneal surgery (Muijzer et al., 2023).

Primary outcome	RD	95%CI
Adverse event rate, unadjusted	0.38	(−9.64–10.64)
Adverse event rate, adjusted for study site	−0.32	(−10.29–9.84)
Separate adverse events:		
Graft detachment, unadjusted	4.64	(−20.08–29.26)
Rebubbling, unadjusted	16.1	(−2.56–37.78)
Graft failure, unadjusted	−2.94	(−15.06–6.34)
Iatrogenic acute glaucoma, unadjusted	−12.03	(−27.27–0.28)

The mean risk difference (RD) and 95% confidence interval (CI) of the outcome measures, and the noninferiority limit (dashed line). The top panel shows the unadjusted and adjusted estimates for the primary outcome measure. The bottom panel shows the unadjusted estimates for all separate postoperative events. For these outcomes, a noninferiority margin is not shown

TABLE 11.9b: Explanation for **Table 11.9a**.

In a noninferiority randomized controlled trial to evaluate the use of intraoperative optical coherence tomography (OCT) during Descemet membrane endothelial keratoplasty, to assess outcomes of the advanced visualization in corneal surgery	
Sample size requirement in noninferiority trial vs. superiority trial is different	The column RD represents the risk difference between two techniques (treatments), and graphical representations of outcome distributions can be used to compare their efficacies. To establish superiority, the outcome graphic should be positioned beyond the noninferiority margin in the zone where the control is deemed better. However, such a study would require a larger sample size, which may present ethical challenges
Source: Muijzer MB, et al.	

$$n = \frac{(k+1)}{k} \frac{\{PQ[Z_{1-\alpha} + Z_{1-\beta}]^2\}}{[|d|-\delta]^2}$$

The quantities $Z_{1-\alpha}$ and $Z_{1-\beta}$ are values from the N (0, 1) corresponding to α and β.
[For $\alpha = 0.05$, $Z_{1-\alpha} = 1.65$ (one-tailed)] **(Tables 11.10a and 11.10b)**
[$Z_{1-\beta}$: Value at specified power ($Z_{0.8} = 0.84$; $Z_{0.9} = 1.28$)]
σ: Pooled standard deviation
d: Anticipated difference in means of the two groups ($\mu_A - \mu_B$)
δ: Margin of clinical significance or testing margin ($\delta < 0$ *for noninferiority and* $\delta > 0$ *for superiority*)
k: Allocation ratio between treatment groups
Note: For a given d, sample sizes increases with higher values of δ.

Sample Size for Equivalence: Comparison of Means

H_1: $-\delta < \mu_A - \mu_B < \delta$ H_1: $|\mu_A - \mu_B| \leq \delta$
Indicates equivalence, which is tested by two one-sided tests.
H_1: $\mu_A - \mu_B < \delta$ and H_1: $\mu_A - \mu_B > -\delta$, where δ is the equivalence margin.

$$n = \frac{(k+1)}{k} \frac{\{\sigma^2[Z_{1-\alpha} + Z_{1-\beta/2}]^2\}}{[|d|-\delta]^2}$$

[$Z_{1-\beta/2}$: Value at specified power ($Z_{0.9} = 1.28$)]

Sample Size for Equivalence: Comparison of two Proportions

H_1: $-\delta < P_A - P_B < \delta$ implies H_1: $P_A - P_B < \delta$
Indicates equivalence, which is tested by two one-sided tests.
H_1: $|P_A - P_B| \leq \delta$ and H_1: $P_A - P_B > -\delta$
Where δ is the equivalence margin.

$$n = \frac{(k+1)}{k} \frac{\{PQ[Z_{1-\alpha} + Z_{1-\beta/2}]^2\}}{[|d|-\delta]^2}$$

$Z_{1-\beta/2}$: Value at specified power ($Z_{0.9} = 1.28$)]

Sequence of Choice

- Before introduction of a new intervention for a particular disease an RCT investigations to evaluate the new intervention can be conducted to check if the new treatment is superior to a placebo control.
- When existence of standard therapy has been established, undertake a placebo-controlled trials: *Unethical.*

- In such situations, *active-controlled trials* can be conducted where a new treatment is compared with an established treatment with the objective of demonstrating that the *new treatment is noninferior*.

Other excellent examples of noninferiority design are illustrated in study titled "Efficacy, durability, and safety of intravitreal faricimab up to every 16 weeks for neovascular age-related macular degeneration (TENAYA and LUCERNE): Two randomized, double-masked, phase 3, noninferiority trials".

It is important to understand that sample size calculation techniques will be different for situations where superiority study was required and the sample requirement will be higher and may pose practical and ethical challenges.

■ CONCLUSION

While placebo-controlled trials are deemed unethical when a standard therapy exists, active-controlled trials can provide valuable insights by comparing new treatments against established ones. Noninferiority trials, such as those evaluating intraoperative OCT during Descemet membrane endothelial keratoplasty and intravitreal faricimab for neovascular age-related macular degeneration, illustrate the importance of these designs. However, these trials require careful consideration of sample size calculations to address ethical and practical challenges.

■ BIBLIOGRAPHY

1. Abdelwhad N, Mohamed M, Yousef H, Mounir A. Clinical outcomes of combined simultaneous femtosecond kerarings implantation and corneal collagen cross-linking in advanced keratoconus. Egypt J Clin Ophthalmol [internet]. 2021 (cited 2021/12/01);4(2):49-55. Available from: https://doi.org/10.21608/ejco.2021.215518
2. Heier JS, Khanani AM, Ruiz CQ, Basu K, Ferrone PJ, Brittain C, et al. Efficacy, durability, and safety of intravitreal faricimab up to every 16 weeks for neovascular age-related macular degeneration (TENAYA and LUCERNE): two randomised, double-masked, phase 3, non-inferiority trials. Lancet [Internet]. 2022 (cited 2022/01/24);399(10326):729-40. Available from: https://doi.org/10.1016/S0140-6736(22)00010-1
3. Li X, Ma W, Song Y, Yap M, Liu L. Comparison of Myopic Progression and Quality of Life Wearing Either DIMs Lenses or Single-Vision Myopia Correcting Spectacles. J Ophthalmol [Internet]. (cited 2025/01/01):2025(1). Available from: https://doi.org/10.1155/joph/9959251
4. Muijzer MB, Delbeke H, Dickman MM, Nuijts RMMA, Noordmans HJ, Imhof SM et al. Frontiers | Outcomes of the advanced visualization in corneal surgery evaluation trial; a non-inferiority randomized control trial to evaluate the use of intraoperative OCT during Descemet membrane endothelial keratoplasty.

Front Ophthalmol [Internet]. 2023 (cited 2023);2. Available from: https://doi.org/10.3389/fopht.2022.1041778

5. Ye Y, Hu Z, Su N, Shen Y, Yuan S. Frontiers | Axial length to corneal curvature radius ratio is negatively correlated with choroidal blood flow in myopic children. Front Ophthalmol [Internet]. 2025 (cited 2025/01/06);4. Available from: https://doi.org/10.3389/fopht.2024.1540410

6. Yousef H, Gad Elkareem A, El Rawy E. Correlation between visual acuity and outer retinal layer thickness in diabetic macular edema. Egypt J Clin Ophthalmol [Internet]. 2024 (cited 2024/12/01);7(2). Available from: https://doi.org/10.21608/ejco.2024.404121

CHAPTER 12

Tools in Data Analysis

Ajay Sharma, T Raveendra, Veerendra Babu Odugu

■ INTRODUCTION

In the rapidly evolving field of data analysis, the right tools can make all the difference. This chapter delves into the essential software and methodologies that empower data analysts to transform raw data into actionable insights. From traditional statistical software to cutting-edge machine learning platforms, we will explore a variety of tools that cater to different aspects of data analysis.

We'll start by examining the foundational tools such as *Excel*, which are indispensable for data manipulation and querying. Next, we have mentioned about more advanced tools like *Python* and *EZR*, which offer robust libraries and frameworks for statistical analysis and data visualization.

By the end of this chapter, you'll have a comprehensive understanding of the tools available for data analysis, their unique features, and how to choose the right tool for your specific needs. Whether you're a beginner looking to get started or an experienced analyst seeking to expand your toolkit, this chapter will provide valuable insights and practical guidance.

■ HOW MS-EXCEL IS TO BE USED WHILE PERFORMING DATA ANALYSIS IN OPHTHALMOLOGY RESEARCH?

Microsoft Excel is a versatile tool that can significantly aid data analysis for ophthalmology research. Its user-friendly interface and powerful features make it accessible to researchers with varying levels of statistical expertise. Here are some ways to utilize MS-Excel in this field:

Data Organization

Excel allows for efficient data entry and organization. Researchers can create spreadsheets to log patient information, treatment details, and outcomes. Features like cell formatting, data validation, and sorting help maintain data integrity and facilitate quick access to specific records.

Descriptive Statistics

Excel's built-in functions enable the calculation of essential descriptive statistics such as mean, median, mode, standard deviation, and range. These statistics provide a preliminary understanding of the data distribution and are crucial for summarizing research findings.

Graphical Representation

Excel offers a variety of charting options such as histograms, scatter plots, line graphs, and bar charts. These visual tools are indispensable for illustrating trends, comparing groups, and presenting data in a comprehensible manner to both academic audiences and laypersons.

Regression Analysis

For more advanced analysis, Excel supports linear regression and other statistical models through its Analysis ToolPak add-in. This can help identify relationships between variables, such as the impact of specific treatments on patient outcomes.

Pivot Tables

Pivot tables are a powerful feature in Excel that allows for dynamic data summarization and exploration. Researchers can quickly aggregate data, find patterns, and conduct subgroup analyses without extensive programming knowledge.

Data Cleaning and Preprocessing

Excel's functions for data cleaning, such as removing duplicates, handling missing values, and performing logical checks, ensure that the dataset is accurate and ready for analysis. This preprocessing step is crucial for obtaining reliable results.

Collaboration and Sharing

Excel files can be easily shared with colleagues, allowing for collaborative analysis. The use of cloud services like OneDrive and SharePoint further facilitates real-time collaboration and version control.

By leveraging these capabilities, ophthalmology researchers can effectively manage and analyze their data, leading to robust and insightful conclusions that advance the field.

Data Analysis in Excel

Enabling the Data Analysis ToolPak

Data Analysis ToolPak is enabled by:
- Open *Excel* and go to the *File* tab.
- Select *Options*.
- In the Excel Options window, select *Add-ins*.
- In the Manage box, select *Excel Add-ins* and click *Go*.
- In the Add-Ins box, check *Analysis ToolPak* (**Figs. 12.1 and 12.2**) and click *OK*.

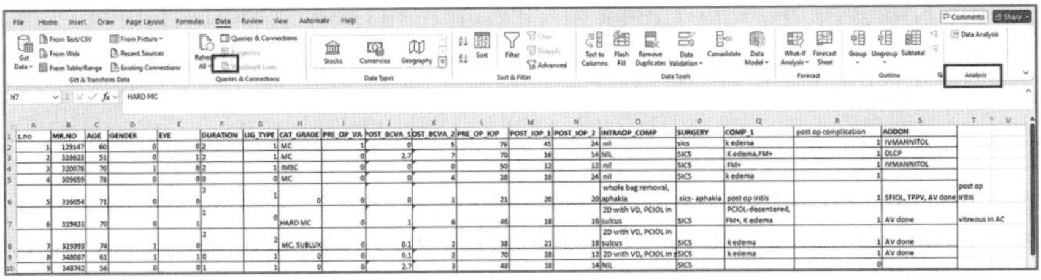

Tools in Data Analysis 163

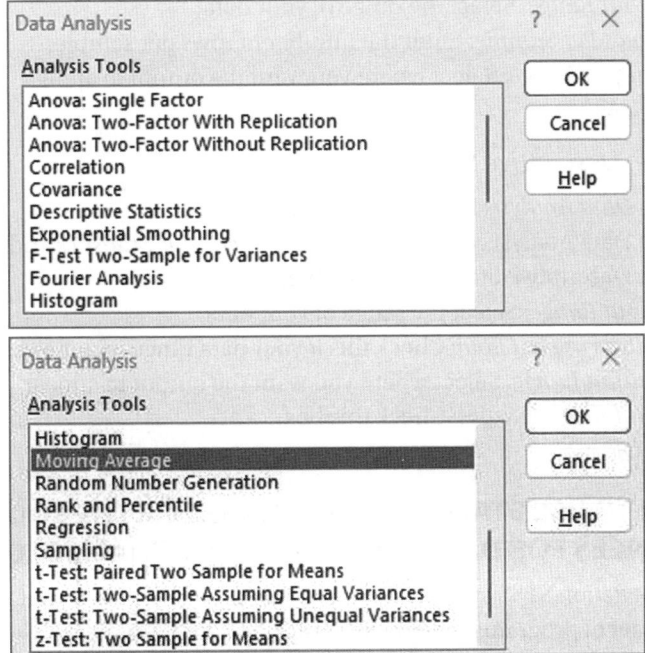

Fig. 12.1: Data representation in Excel and Data Analysis ToolPak representation.

Fig. 12.2: Options available in Data Analysis ToolPak.

Using the Data Analysis Toolpak

Once the ToolPak is enabled, you can access it from the *Data* tab.
- Go to the *Data* tab.
- Click on *Data Analysis* in the Analysis group.
The options available on the Analysis ToolPak are given in **Figure 12.2**:

Example: Performing Analysis of Variance (ANOVA)

Single-factor ANOVA:
- Select *Data Analysis* from the Data tab.
- In the Data Analysis dialog box, select *ANOVA: Single Factor* and click *OK*.
- In the *ANOVA:* Single Factor dialog box:
  - *Input Range:* Select the range of your data.

- *Labels in first row:* Check this if your data range includes labels.
- *Output Range:* Select where you want the output to appear.
■ Click *OK.*

Two-factor ANOVA with replication:
■ Select *Data Analysis* from the Data tab.
■ In the Data Analysis dialog box, select *ANOVA: Two-factor with Replication* and click *OK.*
■ *In the ANOVA:* Two-factor with replication dialog box:
- *Input Range:* Select the range of your data.
- *Rows Per Sample:* Enter the number of rows per sample.
- *Output Range:* Select where you want the output to appear.
■ Click *OK.*

Example: Descriptive Statistics
■ Select *Data Analysis* from the Data tab.
■ In the Data Analysis dialog box, select *Descriptive Statistics* and click *OK.*
■ In the Descriptive Statistics dialog box:
- *Input Range:* Select the range of your data.
- *Labels in First Row:* Check this if your data range includes labels.
- *Output Range:* Select where you want the output to appear.
- *Summary statistics:* Check this box.
■ Click *OK.*

HOW TO USE STATISTICAL PACKAGE FOR THE SOCIAL SCIENCES FOR DATA ANALYSIS IN OPHTHALMOLOGY?

The abbreviation SPSS stands for Statistical Package for the Social Sciences
■ It is a set of programs for data analysis.
■ It was developed for the data analysis needs in the field of Social Science in the year 1968.
■ It is one of widely used programs for statistical analyses.
■ SPSS is widely used in the areas of:
- Health research
- Educational research
- Survey data analysis
- Market research and so on

Using Statistical Package for the Social Sciences

Graphical User Interface (GUI) **(Figs. 12.3 to 12.6):** A point and click approach that is familiar to windows users.
■ For simple analysis with few variables, this approach is mostly used.
■ Many features of SPSS are accessible via pull-down menus.
■ SPSS programming syntax

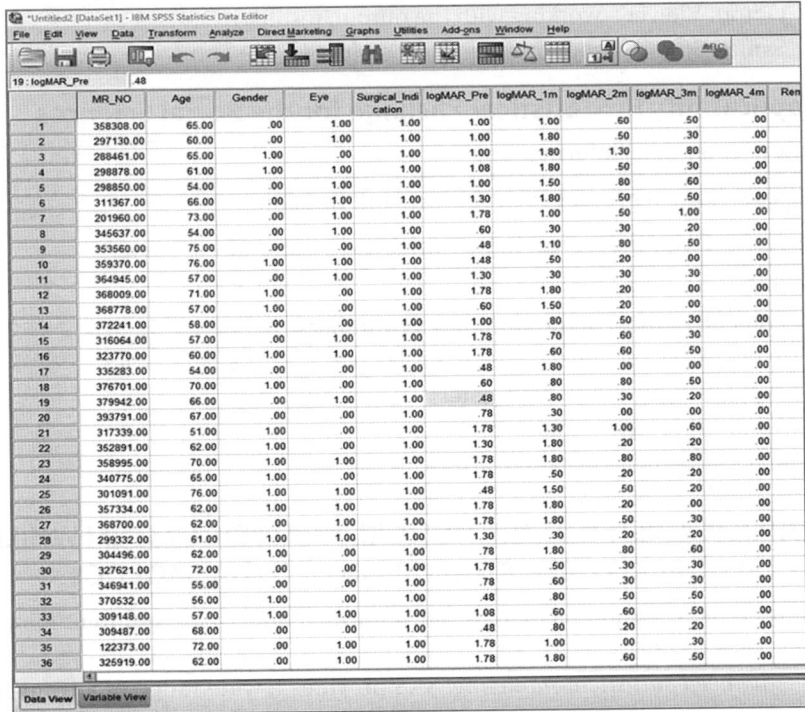

Fig. 12.3: Data representation in Statistical Package for the Social Sciences (SPSS).

A	B	C	D	E	F	G	H	I
SIno	PatientID	Group	Age	AAO	PANSS1	PANSS2	HDRS1	HDRS2
1	12345	Case	26	22	54	77	57	19
2	12346	Control	35	30	58	56	12	14

Fig. 12.4: Correct example of naming a variable in Statistical Package for the Social Sciences (SPSS) tool.

A	B	C	D	E	F	G	H	I
SI#	Patient#	Case/Control	Age	Age@onset	PANSS at Baseline	Followup PANSS score	HDRS1	after Treatment HDRS
1	12345	Case	26	22	54	77	57	19
2	12346	Control	35	30	58	56	12	14

Fig. 12.5: It is advisable not to include special characters (#, $, @) while naming variables in Statistical Package for the Social Sciences (SPSS) tool.

- The command syntax mode is very useful when some set of programs are to be run repeatedly for different subsets of data.
- Some features of SPSS are accessible only via syntax.

Windows in SPSS:
- Data Editor—working with the data:
  - Data View
  - Variable View

- Output Viewer—working with the output/results
- Syntax Editor—programming of procedures

Applicability in Statistical Package for the Social Sciences

How to enter data/information?

Subjects: Rows represent each subject's information.

Variables: Columns represent the variables in the study.

Naming the variables:
- Enter all or most of the variables as numbers
- Avoid using any special characters such as ?, %, *, $, @, <, >, etc.
- Avoid using numbers for names
- Avoid using long phrases
- Maintain uniformity and clarity

APPLICABILITY OF STATISTICAL ANALYSIS SYSTEM WHILE PERFORMING DATA ANALYSIS IN OPHTHALMOLOGY

Using statistical analysis system (SAS) for data analysis in ophthalmology offers several advantages:
- *Advanced statistical modeling:* SAS provides a wide range of advanced statistical modeling techniques that are essential for analyzing complex ophthalmic data, such as paired-eye measurements and longitudinal studies.
- *Handling correlated data:* Ophthalmology research often involves data from both eyes of the same patient, which are typically correlated. SAS has robust methods to handle this correlation, ensuring accurate and reliable results.
- *Data management:* SAS excels in data management, allowing researchers to efficiently handle large datasets, preprocess data, and perform comprehensive analyses. This is particularly useful in clinical trials and genetic studies where data volume and complexity can be high.
- *Customizable and scalable:* SAS is highly customizable and scalable, making it suitable for a wide range of research projects, from small-scale studies to large, multicenter clinical trials.
- *Regulatory compliance:* SAS is widely recognized and accepted by regulatory bodies, making it a preferred choice for clinical trials and other research that requires adherence to strict regulatory standards.
- *Visualization and reporting:* SAS offers powerful tools for data visualization and reporting, helping researchers to present their findings clearly and effectively. This is crucial for communicating results to both scientific and nonscientific audiences.

The SAS user interface is given in **Figure 12.6**.

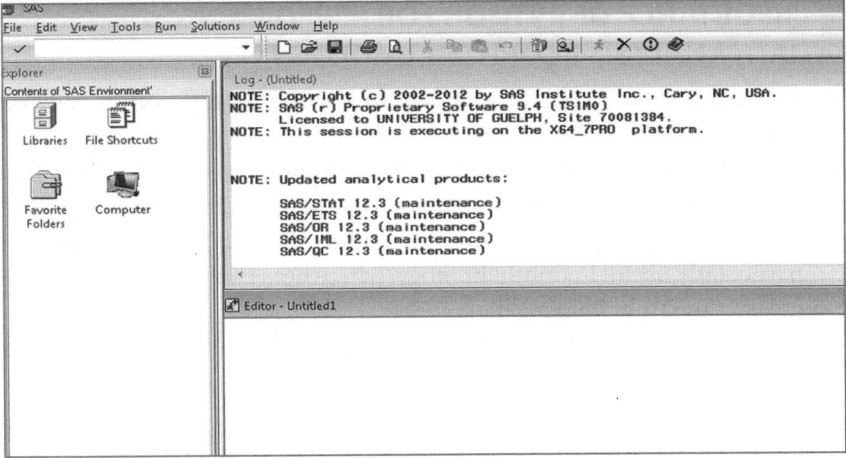

Fig. 12.6: Initial user interface of statistical analysis system (SAS).

USES OF EASY R (EZR) WHILE PERFORMING DATA ANALYSIS IN OPHTHALMOLOGY

Easy R (EZR) is a user-friendly interface for R, a powerful statistical software. It is particularly useful in ophthalmology for several reasons:

- *Accessibility and ease of use:* EZR simplifies the use of R, making it accessible to researchers and clinicians who may not have extensive programming skills. This allows for efficient data analysis without the steep learning curve associated with R.
- *Comprehensive statistical tools:* EZR provides a wide range of statistical tools and tests, from basic descriptive statistics to advanced multivariate analyses. This versatility is beneficial for various types of ophthalmic research, including clinical trials and observational studies.
- *Handling complex data:* Ophthalmology research often involves complex datasets, such as paired-eye data and longitudinal studies. EZR can handle these complexities, allowing for robust statistical analyses.
- *Visualization capabilities:* EZR offers powerful data visualization tools, enabling researchers to create detailed charts, plots, and graphs. This helps in visualizing data trends and patterns, which is crucial for presenting findings clearly.
- *Reproducibility and reliability:* Using EZR ensures that the data analysis process is reproducible and reliable. This is essential for validating research findings and for peer-reviewed publications.
- *Cost-effective:* EZR is free and open source, making it a cost-effective option for researchers and institutions with limited budgets.

By leveraging EZR, ophthalmologists can enhance the accuracy and efficiency of their data analysis, ultimately contributing to better research outcomes and advancements in eye care.

IMPORTANCE OF PYTHON FOR PERFORMING DATA ANALYSIS IN OPHTHALMOLOGY

Using Python for statistical analysis in ophthalmology offers several advantages:

- *Versatility and flexibility:* Python is a versatile programming language that can handle various types of data analysis tasks, from basic descriptive statistics to complex machine-learning models. This flexibility is particularly useful in ophthalmology, where data can range from clinical measurements to imaging data.
- *Extensive libraries:* Python has a rich ecosystem of libraries such as pandas for data manipulation, NumPyn for numerical computations, SciPy for scientific computing, and Stats models for statistical modeling. These libraries provide powerful tools for analyzing ophthalmic data.
- *Data visualization:* Libraries like Matplotlib and Seaborn allow researchers to create detailed and informative visualizations. This is crucial for identifying trends and patterns in ophthalmic data and for presenting findings clearly.
- *Handling large datasets:* Python is capable of efficiently handling large datasets, which is often necessary in ophthalmology research involving extensive patient records or high-resolution imaging data.
- *Reproducibility and transparency:* Python scripts can be easily shared and reproduced, ensuring that analyses are transparent and can be validated by other researchers. This is essential for maintaining the integrity of scientific research.
- *Integration with other tools:* Python can be integrated with other software and tools commonly used in ophthalmology, such as image processing software and electronic health records (EHR) systems. This integration facilitates seamless data analysis workflows.

By leveraging Python, ophthalmologists can enhance the accuracy and efficiency of their data analysis, ultimately contributing to better research outcomes and advancements in eye care.

Tool Epi-Info Use for Data Analysis in Ophthalmology

Using Epi-Info for data analysis in ophthalmology offers several benefits:

- *User-friendly interface:* Epi-Info is designed to be accessible to users without extensive technical backgrounds, making it easier for clinicians and researchers to perform data analysis.
- *Comprehensive statistical tools:* Epi-Info provides a range of statistical tools, including descriptive statistics, regression analysis, and complex sample analysis. These tools are essential for analyzing ophthalmic

data, such as visual acuity measurements and intraocular pressure readings.
- *Data visualization:* Epi-Info includes features for creating maps, graphs, and charts, which help in visualizing data trends and patterns. This is crucial for presenting research findings in a clear and understandable manner.
- *Handling epidemiologic data:* Epi-Info is particularly well-suited for epidemiologic studies, which are common in ophthalmology research. It allows for the analysis of case-control studies, cohort studies, and cross-sectional surveys.
- *Cost-effective:* Epi-Info is free and open-source, making it a cost-effective option for researchers and institutions with limited budgets.

By leveraging Epi-Info, ophthalmologists can enhance the accuracy and efficiency of their data analysis, ultimately contributing to better research outcomes and advancements in eye care.

APPLICATIONS OF G*POWER IN DATA ANALYSIS IN OPHTHALMOLOGY

Using G*Power for data analysis in ophthalmology is highly beneficial for several reasons:
- *Sample size calculation:* G*Power is widely used for determining the appropriate sample size needed for studies. This is crucial in ophthalmology to ensure that studies are adequately powered to detect significant effects, especially when dealing with small or specific patient population **(Figs. 12.7 and 12.8)**.
- *Power analysis:* G*Power allows researchers to perform power analysis, which helps in understanding the likelihood of detecting an effect if it exists. This is important in ophthalmology to design studies that are both efficient and effective.
- *Handling complex study designs:* Ophthalmic studies often involve complex designs, such as paired-eye data or longitudinal studies. G*Power supports various statistical tests (e.g., t-tests, ANOVA, and chi-square tests) and can handle these complexities, ensuring accurate and reliable results.
- *User-friendly interface:* G*Power provides an intuitive interface that simplifies the process of performing sample size and power calculations. This is particularly useful for clinicians and researchers who may not have extensive statistical training.
- *Cost-effective:* G*Power is free and open-source, making it an accessible tool for researchers and institutions with limited budgets.

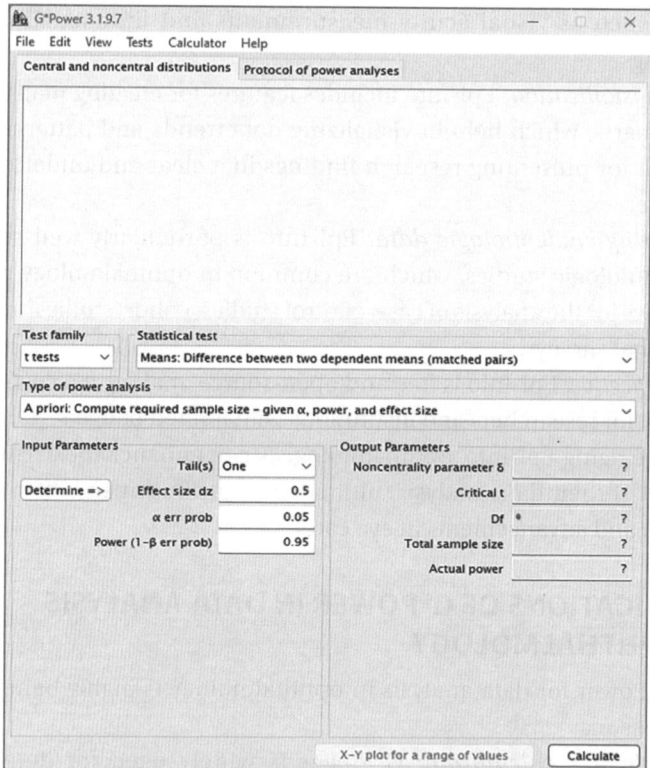

Fig. 12.7: Representing G*power Interface.

By leveraging G*Power, ophthalmologists can enhance the precision and efficiency of their study designs, ultimately contributing to better research outcomes and advancements in eye care.

G*Power Interface is shown in **Figures 12.7 and 12.8**.

ADVANTAGES OF STATA IN STATISTICAL ANALYSIS IN OPHTHALMOLOGY RESEARCH

Using Stata for data analysis in ophthalmology offers several advantages:
- *Advanced statistical methods:* Stata provides a wide range of advanced statistical techniques, including mixed-effects models and generalized estimating equations, which are essential for analyzing correlated eye data.
- *Handling inter-eye correlation:* Ophthalmic data often involves measurements from both eyes of the same patient, which are correlated. Stata has robust methods to account for this correlation, ensuring accurate and reliable results.

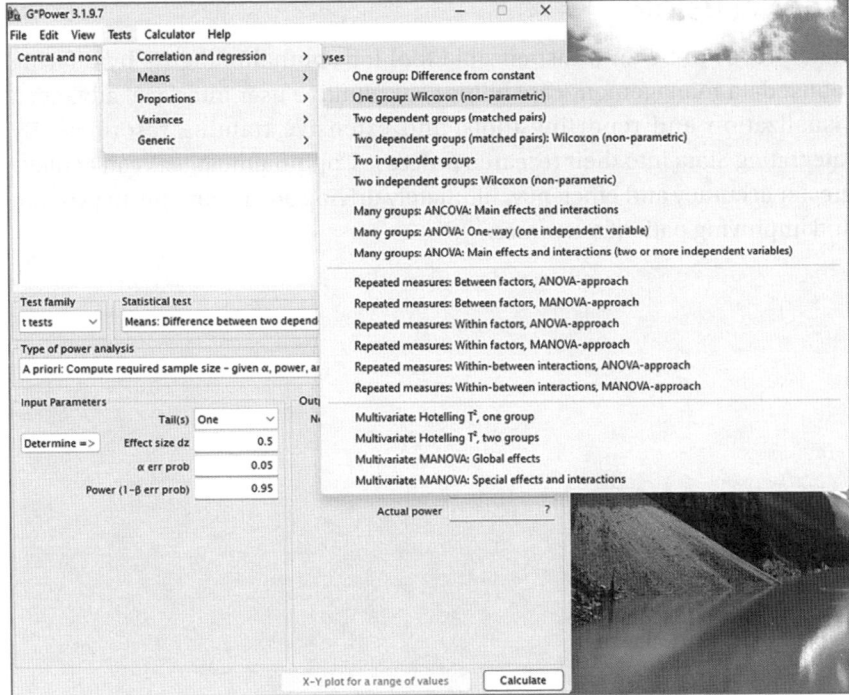

Fig. 12.8: Options available in G*power.

- *Data management:* Stata excels in data management, allowing researchers to efficiently handle large datasets, preprocess data, and perform comprehensive analyses. This is particularly useful in clinical trials and genetic studies where data volume and complexity can be high.
- *User-friendly interface:* Stata offers an intuitive interface that simplifies the process of data entry, manipulation, and analysis. This is particularly beneficial for clinicians and researchers who may not have extensive statistical training.
- *Visualization and reporting:* Stata includes powerful tools for data visualization and reporting, helping researchers to present their findings clearly and effectively. This is crucial for communicating results to both scientific and nonscientific audiences.
- *Training and support:* There are numerous resources available for learning Stata, including online tutorials, courses, and user communities. This support network can help researchers quickly become proficient in using the software.

By leveraging Stata, ophthalmologists can enhance the precision and efficiency of their data analysis, ultimately contributing to better research outcomes and advancements in eye care.

■ CONCLUSION

Stata proves to be an indispensable tool for ophthalmologists by offering robust data management capabilities, an intuitive user interface, advanced visualization and reporting tools, and extensive training resources. By integrating Stata into their research processes, ophthalmologists can achieve greater accuracy and efficiency, ultimately driving advancements in eye care and improving patient outcomes.

CHAPTER 13

Role of Artificial Intelligence in Ophthalmic Statistics

T Raveendra, Manju Valli Pavuluri, B Punyavathi

■ INTRODUCTION

In recent years, the intersection of artificial intelligence (AI) and ophthalmic statistics has emerged as a revolutionary field, promising to transform the landscape of eye care. This chapter aims to provide ophthalmologists with a comprehensive understanding of how AI can be leveraged to enhance statistical analyses in their field, leading to more accurate diagnoses, personalized treatments, and better patient outcomes.

Ophthalmologists, who are often at the forefront of diagnosing and treating complex eye conditions, stand to benefit immensely from the integration of AI into their statistical practices. By automating routine tasks, identifying patterns in large datasets, and offering predictive insights, AI can help clinicians make more informed decisions and streamline their workflow.

Moreover, this chapter will delve into the practical applications of AI in ophthalmic statistics, illustrating how machine learning (ML) models can be trained on vast amounts of clinical data to predict disease progression, assess treatment efficacy, and even uncover new biomarkers for eye diseases.

As we embark on this journey, our goal is to equip you with the essential knowledge and tools to harness the power of AI in your daily practice, ultimately improving the quality of care you provide to your patients.

■ IS MACHINE LEARNING AND ARTIFICIAL INTELLIGENCE RELATED TO STATISTICS IN ANY WAY

Machine learning and AI are closely connected with statistics. Here are several ways they are related:
- *Data analysis:* Statistics enables data analysis, which is an essential step in both ML and AI. Techniques like descriptive statistics help summarize and understand data.
- *Model building:* Many ML algorithms are based on statistical methods. Examples include linear regression, logistic regression, and Bayesian networks, all of which are founded on statistical principles.
- *Probability theory:* This aspect of statistics is widely used in ML and AI for making predictions and handling uncertainty. Algorithms such as Hidden Markov Models (HMM) and Gaussian Mixture Models (GMM) utilize probability theory.

- *Hypothesis testing:* In statistics, hypothesis testing helps make decisions based on data. Similarly, in ML, it assists in evaluating model performance and validating results.

Optimization: Numerous ML and AI techniques depend on optimization, which is a key concept in statistical theory. For instance, gradient descent is an optimization algorithm used to minimize error in ML models.

In summary, statistics provide the theoretical foundation and tools that support the development and operation of ML and AI systems.

Journey from Research Questions to Clinical Applications: Integrating Statistics and Machine Learning/Artificial Intelligence

A typical journey from a research question to its clinical application, incorporating statistics or ML/AI, encompasses several iterative stages, which are discussed here.

Formulating the Research Question

The initial phase involves identifying a specific clinical problem or knowledge gap. The research question should be clear, focused, and feasible. For instance, "Does a new drug reduce the risk of heart attacks in diabetic patients?"

Designing the Study

During this stage, researchers determine the study design (e.g., randomized controlled trial and observational study), population, sample size, and variables to be measured. Statistical tools are employed to calculate the necessary sample size to ensure that the study has adequate power to detect a significant effect.

Data Collection

Data is gathered through various methods such as clinical trials, electronic health records, surveys, or observational studies. Ensuring data quality and consistency is essential for reliable results.

Data Preprocessing

Prior to analysis, data must be cleaned and preprocessed. This includes handling missing values, addressing outliers, and normalizing data. This step ensures that the data is prepared for statistical analysis or ML algorithms.

Data Analysis with Statistics or Machine Learning/Artificial Intelligence

- *Statistics:* Traditional methods such as t-tests, analysis of variance (ANOVA), regression analysis, and hypothesis testing are applied to understand relationships between variables and draw conclusions.
- *ML/AI:* Advanced techniques such as clustering, classification, neural networks, and natural language processing (NLP) are utilized for predictive analytics, pattern recognition, and more.

Interpreting Results

Researchers interpret the analysis results to ascertain whether the research question has been answered. They evaluate the significance, reliability, and applicability of the findings.

Clinical Application

Based on the interpreted results, the findings are translated into clinical practices or recommendations. This includes developing new treatments, enhancing patient care protocols, or informing policy decisions.

Publishing and Peer Review

The findings are documented and submitted to peer-reviewed journals. Peer review ensures the validity and reliability of the research.

Real-World Implementation

Clinical practitioners apply newfound knowledge or treatments in real-world settings. This may involve training healthcare professionals and educating patients.

Continuous Monitoring and Feedback

Postimplementation, the new clinical practices are continuously monitored for effectiveness and safety. Feedback from real-world application often leads to new clinical questions or modifications.

Iteration of the Cycle

New clinical problems and related research questions arise based on feedback and evolving healthcare needs, initiating the cycle anew. This iterative process ensures continual improvement in clinical care.

Example

Consider the identification of a new clinical problem: "Can AI algorithms predict the early onset of sepsis in intensive care unit (ICU) patients?" The process would involve several key steps:

- *Formulating the question:* Clearly define the scope and objectives of the study.
- *Designing the study:* Identify appropriate data sources, determine sample size, and establish methodologies.
- *Data collection:* Collect relevant data from ICU patients.
- *Data preprocessing:* Cleanse and normalize the collected data.
- *ML/AI analysis:* Develop and train predictive algorithms using ML and AI techniques.
- *Interpreting results:* Validate the predictive accuracy of the developed algorithms.
- *Clinical application:* Implement the AI tool within ICU settings.
- *Publishing:* Disseminate findings through medical journals.
- *Real-world implementation:* Apply the AI tool in ICUs and conduct training for healthcare staff.
- *Continuous monitoring:* Continuously monitor the performance of the AI tool and gather user feedback.
- *Iteration:* Refine the AI algorithms based on feedback and address emerging research questions.

This iterative cycle ensures continuous improvement in clinical practices, enhancing the effectiveness and patient-centered nature of healthcare.

ROLE OF ARTIFICIAL INTELLIGENCE IN SUPPORTING STATISTICAL ANALYSIS OF OPHTHALMOLOGICAL STUDIES

Artificial intelligence is rapidly transforming various fields of medicine, and ophthalmology is no exception. The integration of AI into ophthalmological research enhances statistical analysis, enabling more precise, efficient, and comprehensive studies. AI's capabilities in processing vast datasets, identifying intricate patterns, and predicting outcomes are particularly beneficial in the realm of ophthalmology, where large-scale data from diverse sources are often involved.

Enhancing Data Processing and Analysis

Artificial intelligence excels in handling large volumes of data, a common characteristic of ophthalmological studies that include patient records, imaging data, and clinical notes. Advanced AI algorithms can quickly process and analyze these datasets, extracting meaningful insights that might be missed with traditional statistical methods. ML and deep learning, subsets of AI, are particularly adept at recognizing patterns and correlations within complex data, thus providing a more accurate analysis of study results.

Effectiveness in Epidemiological Studies in Ophthalmology

Artificial intelligence technologies enhance epidemiological studies in ophthalmology by processing large datasets and identifying patterns. ML algorithms help uncover relationships within data, providing insights into the prevalence and causes of eye diseases. Deep learning, particularly convolutional neural networks (CNNs), improve the analysis of medical images, aiding in the early detection of conditions like diabetic retinopathy and glaucoma.

Natural language processing extracts valuable information from electronic medical records (EMRs) and clinical notes, identifying patients at risk for various eye diseases. Predictive modeling, based on historical data, helps forecast the onset and progression of eye diseases, enabling timely intervention.

Artificial intelligence-powered telemedicine platforms facilitate remote screening and diagnosis, making eye care more accessible. These innovations enhance the statistical robustness of epidemiological studies, ensuring representative and applicable findings.

Machine Learning Algorithms

Machine learning algorithms, such as decision trees, random forests, and support vector machines, are employed to analyze large datasets, identifying patterns and relationships that contribute to disease understanding and treatment strategies. For instance, random forests can predict the risk of developing conditions like diabetic retinopathy based on a patient's health data.

Deep Learning Algorithms

Deep learning, and more specifically CNNs, play a crucial role in medical image analysis. These algorithms can detect subtle abnormalities in retinal images with high accuracy, facilitating early diagnosis and intervention. The ability of CNNs to process and learn from extensive imaging data enhances the statistical analysis of visual health studies, providing robust and reliable results.

■ NATURAL LANGUAGE PROCESSING

Natural language processing is another AI technology that supports ophthalmology by extracting relevant information from unstructured text data, such as EMRs and clinical notes. NLP algorithms can analyze these documents to identify patients at risk for various eye diseases, thus aiding in the creation of comprehensive and data-driven study analyses.

Natural language processing has emerged as a transformative technology in various fields, including health care. In ophthalmology, NLP can significantly enhance the process of data collection from case records, revolutionizing how patient information is gathered, analyzed, and utilized.

Understanding Natural Language Processing

Natural language processing is a branch of AI that focuses on the interaction between computers and human language. It enables machines to understand, interpret, and generate human language, facilitating the extraction of valuable information from unstructured text data such as EMRs and clinical notes.

Data Collection Challenges

Traditional methods of data collection from case records often involve manual data entry and review, which can be time-consuming, error-prone, and inconsistent. The vast amount of unstructured data within case records, such as physician notes, diagnostic reports, and patient histories, poses significant challenges for efficient and accurate data collection.

How Natural Language Processing Enhances Data Collection

Natural language processing addresses these challenges by automating the extraction of relevant information from unstructured text data. Here are several ways NLP can be beneficial.

Automated Data Extraction

Natural language processing algorithms can automatically extract key information from clinical notes, such as patient demographics, medical history, symptoms, diagnoses, and treatment plans. This automation reduces the need for manual data entry, saving time and reducing the risk of human error.

Identification of At-risk Patients

By analyzing case records, NLP can identify patients at risk for various eye diseases. For example, it can detect mentions of early symptoms or risk factors for the conditions like diabetic retinopathy or glaucoma, allowing for timely intervention and improved patient outcomes.

Improved Data Consistency

Natural language processing ensures data consistency by standardizing the extraction process. It can recognize and normalize different terminologies and abbreviations used by various healthcare providers, ensuring that the data collected is uniform and comparable across different records.

Enhanced Data Analysis

Natural language processing facilitates the analysis of large datasets by extracting structured information from unstructured text. This structured data can then be used for statistical analysis, epidemiological studies, and predictive modeling, providing deeper insights into the prevalence and progression of eye diseases.

Case Study: Ophthalmology

In ophthalmology, NLP has shown promising results in extracting valuable information from EMRs. For instance, NLP algorithms can analyze clinical notes to identify patients with early signs of diabetic retinopathy, enabling early intervention. Similarly, by extracting data from visual field test reports, NLP can help monitor the progression of glaucoma and adjust treatment plans accordingly.

Conclusion

Natural language processing is a powerful tool that can revolutionize data collection from case records in ophthalmology. By automating the extraction of relevant information, identifying at-risk patients, ensuring data consistency, and enhancing data analysis, NLP contributes to more efficient and accurate data collection. As the technology continues to evolve, its integration into healthcare practices will undoubtedly lead to improved patient care and research outcomes.

ARTIFICIAL INTELLIGENCE TOOLS FOR STATISTICAL ANALYSIS, COMPARISON WITH STATISTICAL PACKAGE FOR THE SOCIAL SCIENCES

Features:
- *Statistical Package for the Social Sciences (SPSS):* Focuses on traditional statistical analysis, offering tools for descriptive statistics, inferential statistics, and various forms of regression analysis.
- *AI tools:* Provide advanced ML and deep learning capabilities, enabling more complex and nuanced data analysis.

Flexibility:
- *SPSS:* Uses predefined procedures and requires manual coding for custom analyses.
- *AI tools:* Offer greater flexibility with dynamic computational graphs (PyTorch), modular approaches (KNIME), and user-friendly interfaces (RapidMiner).

Scalability:
- *SPSS:* Suitable for small to medium-sized datasets but may struggle with very large datasets.
- *AI tools:* Designed to handle large-scale data processing and complex neural network architectures, making them ideal for big data applications.

Usability:
- *SPSS:* Requires knowledge of statistical methods and manual coding for advanced analyses.
- *AI Tools:* Many offer intuitive, user-friendly interfaces (e.g., RapidMiner) and support for nonprogrammers.

Integration:
- *SPSS:* Primarily a standalone tool with limited integration capabilities.
- *AI Tools:* Often part of larger ecosystems (e.g., TensorFlow with Google Cloud, Watson with IBM Cloud) and can be easily integrated with other data science workflows.

Conclusion

While SPSS remains a powerful tool for traditional statistical analysis, AI tools provide enhanced capabilities for handling complex data and performing advanced analytics. Tools like TensorFlow, PyTorch, RapidMiner, KNIME, and IBM Watson offer greater flexibility, scalability, and integration options, making them suitable for modern data science applications. As the field of AI continues to evolve, these tools are likely to become increasingly important in the landscape of statistical analysis.

IMPACT OF ARTIFICIAL INTELLIGENCE AND MACHINE LEARNING TOOLS ON RESEARCH METHODOLOGIES IN OPHTHALMOLOGY

Artificial intelligence and ML are transforming the landscape of ophthalmic research, introducing innovative methodologies and enhancing the precision of statistical analysis. As these technologies continue to evolve, researchers and practitioners must adapt to new paradigms in data collection, analysis, and interpretation.

Data Collection and Preprocessing

Artificial intelligence and ML tools necessitate high-quality, large-scale datasets for accurate model training. As a result, research methodologies are shifting toward comprehensive data collection practices, ensuring diverse and representative samples. Automated data preprocessing techniques, such as image enhancement and normalization, are becoming standard, leading to more efficient and reliable data preparation.

Algorithm Development and Training

The advent of AI and ML has introduced the need for developing and training complex algorithms tailored to ophthalmic data. Researchers are now focusing on creating robust models capable of handling the intricacies of medical images and patient records. This includes selecting appropriate algorithms for specific tasks, such as CNNs for image analysis or recurrent neural networks for time-series data.

Statistical Analysis and Interpretation

Traditional statistical methods are being augmented with AI-driven approaches, enabling the extraction of deeper insights from ophthalmic data. ML algorithms can uncover hidden patterns and correlations that may be missed by conventional techniques. Researchers are now employing predictive modeling, data mining, and other advanced methods to enhance the accuracy and reliability of their findings.

Integration of Multimodal Data

Artificial intelligence and ML facilitate the integration of multimodal data, combining information from various sources such as retinal images, genetic data, and clinical records. This holistic approach allows for a more comprehensive understanding of ocular diseases and their progression. Researchers are developing methodologies to seamlessly integrate and analyze these diverse datasets, leading to more informed and personalized treatment strategies.

Ethical Considerations and Bias Mitigation

The use of AI in ophthalmic research raises important ethical considerations, including data privacy, informed consent, and potential biases in algorithm development. Researchers must adopt methodologies that prioritize patient confidentiality and address biases that may arise from unbalanced training data. Transparent reporting and validation practices are essential to ensure the ethical use of AI tools.

Continuous Learning and Adaptation

Artificial intelligence and ML models require continuous learning and adaptation to remain effective. Researchers are developing methodologies for ongoing model validation and updating, incorporating new data and feedback to improve performance. This dynamic approach ensures that AI-driven tools remain relevant and accurate in the face of evolving medical knowledge and practices.

■ CONCLUSION

The integration of AI and ML tools is revolutionizing research methodologies in ophthalmology, offering unprecedented opportunities for innovation and precision. As researchers and practitioners embrace these technologies, they must adapt to new paradigms in data collection, algorithm development, and ethical considerations. By staying at the forefront of AI-driven advancements, the ophthalmic community can pave the way for a new era of precision medicine and improved patient outcomes.

■ BIBLIOGRAPHY

1. Friedrich S, Antes G, Behr S, Binder H, Brannath W, Dumpert F, et al. Is there a role for statistics in artificial intelligence? Adv Data Anal Classif [Internet]. 2022 (cited 06/08/2021);16:823-46. Available from: https://link.springer.com/article/10.1007/s11634-021-00455-6
2. Hirani R, Noruzi K, Khuram H, Hussaini AS, Aifuwa EI, Ely KE, et al. Artificial Intelligence and Healthcare: A Journey through History, Present Innovations, and Future Possibilities. Life (Basel) [Internet]. 2024(cited 2024 Apr);14(5):557. Available from: https://pmc.ncbi.nlm.nih.gov/articles/PMC11122160/
3. Santos Arteaga FJ, Di Caprio D, Tavana M, Cucchiari D, Campistol JM, Oppenheimer F, et al. On the capacity of artificial intelligence techniques and statistical methods to deal with low-quality data in medical supply chain environment. Eng Appl Artif Intell [Internet]. 2024 (cited 2024 July);133 (Part F): 108610. Available from: https://www.sciencedirect.com/science/article/pii/S0952197624007681

CHAPTER 14

Collaboration with Biostatistician

Krishna Talabhaktula, Kavithadevi Mamchimsetti, B Punyavathi

▉ INTRODUCTION

Effective communication with a statistician is crucial for the success of any data-driven project in ophthalmology. This chapter outlines a comprehensive plan for such communication, detailing when to reach out, what information to provide, and the formats of queries. Clear and timely interactions ensure that the statistician can offer the best support, from the initial stages of project planning through to the analysis and interpretation of results.

For ophthalmologists, whether residents or consultants, it is important to establish a timeline for engaging with a statistician. Early contact is recommended when conceptualizing a study or planning an implementation project. This initial interaction should include a detailed overview of your research question or hypothesis, the specific aims of your study, and any preliminary data you might have.

▉ INFORMATION FOR STATISTICIAN

Providing the statistician with detailed information from the outset is critical for several reasons. Firstly, it ensures that the statistician has a clear understanding of the research objectives and study design, which allows them to offer the most appropriate statistical methods and analyses tailored to your project. Secondly, by sharing comprehensive data collection methods and variables, you help the statistician identify potential challenges and confounders early on, thereby minimizing errors and enhancing the reliability of your results. Thirdly, clear communication of your research questions and aims allows the statistician to align their support with your project's goals, leading to more insightful interpretations and robust conclusions. Ultimately, this collaboration facilitates smooth workflow, reduces the risk of miscommunication, and enhances the overall quality and impact of the research, benefiting both the ophthalmologists and their patients.

- *Research objective:* Clearly state the purpose of your study and its significance in the field of ophthalmology.
- *Study design:* Describe the type of study (e.g., randomized controlled trial, cohort study, case–control study) and the rationale behind choosing this design.
- *Data collection methods:* Explain how data will be gathered, including details on sample size, inclusion/exclusion criteria, and the types of data

to be collected (e.g., visual acuity measurements, intraocular pressure readings, and imaging results).
- *Variables and outcomes:* Identify the primary and secondary outcomes you aim to investigate as well as any independent variables and potential confounders.

■ CLARITY AND CONCISENESS IN QUERIES

- *Email:* Use structured emails with specific subject lines and bullet points to outline your questions and data needs.
- *Meetings:* Schedule regular meetings, either in-person or virtually, to discuss progress and address any emerging issues.
- *Documentation:* Maintain detailed records of all communications and decisions made, which can be referenced throughout the project.

By understanding the optimal times to contact the statistician and the specific information they require, ophthalmologists can facilitate smooth and productive collaboration. This will ultimately enhance the quality and impact of their research or implementation projects, leading to better patient outcomes and advancements in the field of ophthalmology.

▌ PHASES OF A PROJECT OR STUDY AND COLLABORATION NEEDS

Effective communication is a cornerstone of successful project management. Whether you are working with a small team or coordinating efforts across multiple departments, clear and consistent communication plays a crucial role in ensuring that everyone comprehends their roles, responsibilities, and the project's overarching objectives. Effective communication helps prevent misunderstandings, promotes collaboration, and ensures that all team members are moving in the same direction toward common goals.

This chapter outlines the key phases of a project and highlights the essential communication needed at each stage. By understanding these phases and implementing the recommended communication strategies, project managers can facilitate smoother workflows, enhance team cohesion, and increase the likelihood of meeting project deadlines and achieving desired outcomes.

Clear communication with statisticians and staff is particularly vital for the success of any project involving data collection and analysis. Proper communication ensures that statistical methods are appropriately designed and implemented, data integrity is maintained, and the results are accurately interpreted and disseminated to all stakeholders. This chapter explains the various phases of a project and the specific communication requirements at each stage, providing a roadmap for effective project execution from inception to completion.

Planning Phase

The planning phase is a critical stage where the foundation of the research is established. Clear and consistent communication with the statistician is essential during this phase. Key elements to address include:

Research Objective

In this phase, it is imperative to clearly articulate the purpose of the study and its significance. Effective communication with the statistician should encompass:
- A comprehensive description of the research objective, including specific aims and hypotheses
- An explanation of its importance in the field of ophthalmology, addressing how it will fill existing gaps in knowledge or practice
- Iterative meetings within the research team under guidance of leadership, to refine objectives and ensure they are measurable and achievable.

Literature Review

Additionally, holding journal presentations or journal clubs to study similar studies can be immensely beneficial. These forums allow the team to:
- *Review limitations:* Understand the limitations faced by other studies, which can help in designing a more robust study
- *Explore new visualizations:* Discuss potential new visualizations and methodologies that could be applied to the current study to improve data interpretation and presentation

By examining similar studies and existing data and through active engagement in journal presentations and clubs, the team can establish the most appropriate sample size, inclusion and exclusion criteria, and the types of data to be collected. This will enhance the robustness of the study design and increase the likelihood of obtaining valid and reliable results.

Study Design

Describe the type of study and justify the chosen design. Discuss with the statistician to ensure alignment with your research objectives. Key points to address include:
- Type of study (e.g., randomized controlled trial, cohort study, and case-control study) and the rationale for selecting this design
- Detailed methodology, including sampling methods, data collection techniques, and tools to be used (e.g., visual acuity measurements, intraocular pressure readings, and imaging results)
- Potential sources of bias and strategies to mitigate them

- Inclusion and exclusion criteria for participant selection to ensure a representative sample that can provide reliable and valid results.

Nature of Main Data

Explain how data will be gathered, including details on sample size, inclusion/exclusion criteria, and the types of data to be collected. Points to consider:
- Visual acuity measurements using standard tests like the Snellen chart or Early Treatment Diabetic Retinopathy Study (ETDRS) chart
- Intraocular pressure readings using devices such as Goldmann applanation tonometry or noncontact tonometry
- Imaging results from techniques like optical coherence tomography (OCT), fundus photography, or fluorescein angiography.

Variables and Outcomes

Identify the primary and secondary outcomes you aim to investigate as well as any independent variables and potential confounders:
- Primary outcomes might include changes in visual acuity, reduction in intraocular pressure, or improvement in retinal thickness.
- Secondary outcomes could involve quality-of-life assessments, patient satisfaction, or adherence to treatment protocols.
- Independent variables may include demographic factors, baseline clinical characteristics, or treatment modalities.
- Confounders to consider might be comorbid conditions, concurrent medications, or environmental factors.

Sample Size Calculation

At this stage, it is crucial for the researcher and the statistician to engage in detailed discussions regarding the sample size. This collaborative effort should involve a thorough review of the published literature in the area to identify trends, methodologies, and results from similar studies. By doing so, they can ensure that the sample size is adequately powered to detect meaningful differences and to account for variability within the collected data.

Key points to consider in these discussions include:
- *Inclusion and exclusion criteria:* Define criteria clearly to select a representative sample while minimizing bias. This may include specific demographic factors, clinical characteristics, or other relevant variables.
- *Types of data to be collected:* Visual acuity measurements using standard tests like the Snellen chart or ETDRS (LogMAR) chart, intraocular pressure readings using devices such as Goldmann applanation tonometry or

noncontact tonometry, and imaging results from techniques like OCT, fundus photography, or fluorescein angiography.

Utilize statistical techniques to determine the minimum number of participants needed to achieve significant results, considering the expected effect size, power, and significance level.

Scientific Committee Rigor

The scientific committee assesses the scientific merit and feasibility of the proposed study. Their review focuses on the following aspects:

- *Study rationale:* The committee ensures that the study addresses a significant gap or question in the field of ophthalmology. They evaluate the background and justification for the study, examining whether the research is built on a solid foundation of existing knowledge and whether it aims to advance understanding in a meaningful way.
- *Methodological rigor:* They scrutinize the proposed study design and methods, including the study's objectives, hypotheses, and statistical analyses. The committee considers whether the methodologies are appropriate for achieving the research aims, whether the study is sufficiently powered to detect meaningful effects, and whether potential confounders and biases are adequately addressed.
- *Feasibility:* The committee reviews the practical aspects of the study, such as the proposed timeline, the availability of resources (including funding, equipment, and personnel), and potential logistical challenges. They assess whether the study can be completed within the projected timeframe and budget and whether the research team has the necessary expertise and experience to carry out the study successfully.

Ethics Committee Rigor

The ethics committee evaluates the ethical considerations of the proposed study to protect participants' rights and well-being. Their review includes:

- *Informed consent:* Ensuring that the process for obtaining informed consent from participants is thorough and comprehensible, detailing the study's purpose, procedures, risks, and benefits, and confirming that participants have the opportunity to ask questions and withdraw at any time
- *Risk–Benefit analysis:* Assessing whether the potential benefits of the study outweigh the risks involved for participants, considering both short-term and long-term impacts on participants' health and well-being
- *Confidentiality:* Reviewing how sensitive data will be protected, ensuring compliance with relevant data protection regulations such as General Data Protection Regulation (GDPR), and outlining methods for securely storing and sharing data to prevent unauthorized access

- *Vulnerable populations:* Providing special consideration for studies involving vulnerable groups (e.g., children, elderly, or those with cognitive impairments), ensuring additional protections are in place to safeguard their participation and well-being.

The specific role of the statistician in this context is crucial. The statistician provides expertise in:
- *Study design:* Advising on the appropriate study design and statistical methodologies to ensure the study is robust and capable of addressing the research questions effectively
- *Sample size calculation:* Determining the optimal sample size needed to achieve reliable and valid results, ensuring the study is sufficiently powered to detect meaningful differences or effects
- *Data analysis plan:* Developing a comprehensive data analysis plan, including specifying statistical tests to be used, handling missing data, and addressing potential confounders
- *Interim analysis:* Conducting interim analyses to monitor the study's progress, identify any emerging issues, and advise on potential modifications to the study protocol to enhance its validity and reliability
- *Final data analysis:* Performing the final data analysis, interpreting the results, and assisting in the preparation of reports and manuscripts for publication.

Data Collection Phase

Data Collection Methods

Data collection involves various methodologies to ensure comprehensive and accurate gathering of information. The primary methods include:
- *Surveys and questionnaires:* These involve utilizing structured forms to collect standardized information from participants. This method is efficient for collecting large amounts of data quickly.
- *Interviews:* These involve conducting face-to-face, telephonic, or virtual interviews to gather in-depth information and insights from participants. Interviews can be structured, semi-structured, or unstructured.
- *Observations:* These involve directly observing and recording behaviors, events, or conditions as they occur. This method is particularly useful for capturing real-time data in natural settings.
- *Medical and clinical tests:* Administering various tests and procedures to collect physiological and clinical data, such as blood tests, imaging studies, and physical examinations.
- *Use of electronic health records (EHRs):* Extracting relevant data from digital health records to obtain comprehensive patient information, including medical history, treatment plans, and outcomes.

- *Focus groups:* These include facilitating group discussions to explore participants' perceptions, opinions, and attitudes toward a particular topic. This method is useful for gaining qualitative insights.
- *Sensor-based data collection:* Utilizing wearable devices and sensors to continuously monitor and collect data on various physiological parameters, such as heart rate, activity levels, and sleep patterns.

Collection Process

During this phase, regular updates on data collection progress and any encountered issues are essential. The communication should include:

- *Structured emails with updates and queries:* Send detailed emails summarizing the progress, challenges, and any deviations from the protocol.
- *Regular meetings (in-person or virtual) to discuss progress:* Schedule bi-weekly or monthly meetings to review collected data, address concerns, and ensure everything is on track.
- *Detailed documentation of communications and decisions:* Maintain a comprehensive log of all communications, decisions made, and any changes to the study plan to ensure transparency and accountability.

Data verification and validation: Implement procedures to verify and validate the data collected to ensure its accuracy, completeness, and reliability.

Data security and confidentiality: Ensure that all collected data is stored securely and that confidentiality protocols are strictly followed to protect participant information. This includes implementing encryption for data storage and transfer, restricting access to authorized personnel only, and regularly auditing security practices to prevent breaches.

Anonymization protocols: To further protect participant privacy, employ anonymization techniques such as removing or masking personal identifiers from the dataset. This may involve assigning unique codes to each participant, aggregating data to a level that prevents individual identification, and using specialized software to ensure that data cannot be traced back to individuals. Additionally, establish clear guidelines on how and when anonymized data can be shared or published, ensuring compliance with ethical standards and regulations.

Backup and data storage solutions: Develop a robust backup and storage plan to prevent data loss and facilitate easy retrieval of information as needed.

Training and support for data collectors: Provide ongoing training and support to individuals involved in data collection to ensure consistency and quality in data-gathering methods.

Data Analysis Phase

Preliminary Analysis

Once data collection is complete, the next step involves conducting a preliminary analysis. This initial review aims to identify any anomalies, inconsistencies, or unexpected trends within the dataset. Effective communication during this phase is crucial and should include:

- *Prompt sharing of preliminary results:* The preliminary findings should be promptly shared with the statistician and other key team members. This ensures that any potential issues are identified and addressed early.
- *Discussion of anomalies:* Any anomalies or trends observed during this initial analysis should be thoroughly discussed. These discussions may involve identifying potential sources of error, considering additional variables, or adjusting the analysis approach.

Final Analysis

During the final analysis phase, detailed statistical analyses are performed to test the study's hypotheses. This phase requires meticulous attention to detail and ongoing communication to ensure the accuracy and integrity of the findings. Key communication needs include:

- *Clear presentation of analysis results:* The results of the final analysis should be presented clearly and systematically. This presentation should include comprehensive statistical tables, graphs, and figures that accurately represent the data.
- *Frequent consultations to interpret findings:* Regular consultations with the statistician and other experts are essential to interpret the findings accurately. These consultations help in understanding the clinical significance of the results and in making data-driven decisions about the study's conclusions.

Reporting Phase

Manuscript Preparation

The preparation of the manuscript is a critical step in the reporting phase. It involves detailing your study findings with precision and clarity to ensure they are comprehensible and impactful. Statisticians play a vital role at this stage by assisting with the interpretation of results and the preparation of statistical tables and figures. Effective communication during this phase should include:

- *Structured drafts shared for review:* Circulate well-organized drafts of the manuscript among your team members, particularly the statistician, for their input and review. This ensures that the data is accurately represented and that any potential errors are identified and corrected early in the process.

- *Regular feedback sessions:* Schedule regular meetings or feedback sessions to discuss the drafts. These discussions provide an opportunity to address any questions or concerns, refine the analysis, and enhance the overall quality of the manuscript.

Submission and Publication

Once the manuscript is finalized, the next step is submission for publication. This involves adhering to the guidelines of the target journal and ensuring that all communications with the statistician and supporting staff are meticulously documented. Key communication needed at this stage include:

- *Final review of the manuscript:* Conduct a thorough final review of the manuscript, focusing on the accuracy and clarity of the statistical analyses and the presentation of the data. This review should involve both the ophthalmologist and the statistician to ensure that all aspects of the study are comprehensively covered.
- *Documentation of all communications:* Maintain detailed records of all communications related to the manuscript preparation and submission process. This documentation is essential for tracking progress, managing resources, and ensuring accountability. It also provides a reference for any future queries or follow-up actions.

Postpublication Phase

Dissemination of Results

After the manuscript has been finalized and accepted for publication, the next crucial step is the dissemination of your study results to the broader ophthalmology community. This can be achieved through various channels, such as conferences, seminars, and peer-reviewed journals. Statisticians can provide invaluable assistance by conducting additional analyses if required or by helping to draft responses to any reviewer's comments. Effective communication at this stage should include:

- *Structured emails with dissemination plans:* Detailed emails outlining the specific plans for disseminating the results, including target journals, conferences, and any other relevant forums
- *Meetings to discuss additional analyses or responses:* Regularly scheduled meetings to discuss any further statistical analyses needed or to formulate comprehensive responses to queries from reviewers or the scientific community.

Ongoing Collaboration

Maintaining open lines of communication with statisticians and supporting staff is essential for fostering future research opportunities. This ongoing

collaboration can lead to new projects and further advancements in the field of ophthalmology. Key aspects of this phase include:
- *Regular check-ins to discuss potential projects:* Schedule periodic meetings to brainstorm and discuss potential new research projects, ensuring that all team members are aligned and informed.
- *Documentation of ongoing collaborations:* Keep detailed records of all communications and collaborative efforts. This documentation is vital for tracking progress, managing resources, and maintaining accountability.

CONCLUSION

By understanding the specific communication needs at each phase of a project or study, researchers can ensure smooth and productive collaboration with statisticians and supporting staff. This will ultimately enhance the quality and impact of their research, leading to better patient outcomes and advancements in the field of ophthalmology.

APPENDICES

APPENDIX 1

Research Frameworks in Clinical Ophthalmology

T Raveendra, B Muniswami

■ INTRODUCTION

In the intricate world of clinical ophthalmology, research frameworks serve as the backbone for generating new knowledge and improving patient outcomes. This chapter delves into the essential components of research methodology, providing a structured approach to designing and conducting studies. From formulating hypotheses to selecting appropriate study designs, each step is crucial in ensuring the validity and reliability of the research findings. By understanding and applying these frameworks, ophthalmologists can contribute to evidence-based practice and advance the field of eye care.

To build a robust research framework in clinical ophthalmology, it is imperative to comprehend several foundational aspects. These include the study objective, which defines the focus of the research; the study design, which outlines the methodology; and the study population, which specifies the demographic or clinical group under investigation. Understanding these elements is crucial for minimizing bias, ensuring the validity and reliability of the data, and ultimately contributing meaningful insights to the field. By meticulously addressing each of these components, researchers can lay a solid groundwork for their studies, facilitating the advancement of ophthalmic practices and patient care.

Study Objective

What do we want to know or study? Frame this as a hypothesis. This might involve asking specific questions about a topic of interest, such as "Does a new teaching method improve student performance?" or "What are the effects of a particular diet on overall health?" Clearly defining the study objective helps in narrowing down the focus and establishing the purpose of the research.

Study Designs

Base this on the study objective or hypothesis. Consider what type of data will be collected and how it will be analyzed. For instance, if the objective is to examine the impact of a new drug, the study might use a randomized controlled trial (RCT) to compare outcomes between a treatment group and a control group. The design should detail the methodology, including sample size, selection criteria, data collection procedures, and statistical methods to ensure reliable and valid results.

Study designs have been described in detail later in this chapter with a flow chart for easier understanding of the concept **Flowchart 1.1**.

Study Population

After framing the hypothesis and designing the study, it is necessary to identify the population from which study participants will be drawn. This target population, where the pattern or prevalence, or incidence of the disease or outcomes of the intervention will be studied, forms the study population. The population can consist of animate or inanimate objects; however, in the context of medical science or ophthalmology, the population is always animate.

Before further proceeding into study designs, let us get introduced to a few more important concepts of biostatistics.

Bias

Bias refers to systematic errors that affect the validity of research findings. It can occur during study design, data collection, data analysis, and interpretation, leading to incorrect or misleading conclusions.

Types of bias include selection bias **(Table 1.1)**, information bias **(Table 1.2)**, and confounding bias **(Table 1.3)**. Selection bias happens when study participants are not representative of the target population. Information bias arises from measurement or data collection errors. Confounding occurs when an external variable influences both the independent and dependent variables.

TABLE 1.1: Selection bias was represented in this article.	
Selection bias: "Correlation between visual acuity and outer retinal layer thickness in diabetic macular edema"	
Selection bias	Selection bias can arise in studied cases with macular edema not due to diabetic retinopathy, such as subretinal fluid in cystoid macular edema, retinal vein occlusion, postinflammatory, or postsurgical edema

TABLE 1.2: Information bias was reduced by restricting a less than one-year gap in selecting study subjects.	
Information bias was reduced in "Immediate sequential versus delayed sequential bilateral cataract surgery: retrospective comparison of postoperative visual outcomes."	
Information bias	We included patients who had undergone an operation in both eyes for cataract within one year. We did not include patients who had a gap of more than one year between cataract surgeries to restrict information bias about the number of hospital visits and optometry services required

TABLE 1.3: Confounding bias was eliminated by removing faulty studies in the meta-analysis.	
Confounding bias was found in "Associations of statin use with the onset and progression of open-angle glaucoma: A systematic review and meta-analysis."	
Confounding bias	Potential risks of bias were detected in 12 studies, which were then excluded from the meta-analysis, mainly to reduce statistical error in the meta-analysis attributed to selection and confounding bias

Minimizing bias is essential for reliable research findings. Methods to reduce bias include randomization, blinding, proper study design, and rigorous data collection and analysis techniques.

Blinding

Blinding is a technique used in research to prevent bias by concealing the group allocation from one or more parties involved in the study. The goal is to ensure that expectations or knowledge about the intervention do not influence the participants, researchers, or those analyzing the data.

There are several types of blinding:
- *Single-blind:* In this type, the participants do not know which group (control or treatment) they are in, but the researchers do.
- *Double-blind:* Both the participants and the researchers conducting the study are unaware of the group allocations. This method is particularly effective in reducing bias **(Table 1.4)**.

TABLE 1.4: Double blinding in research to reduce bias.	
Double blinding: "Ologen implant versus mitomycin C for trabeculectomy: A systematic review and meta-analysis"	
Double blinding	In this study, both the participants and the investigator were blinded to reduce selection bias.

- *Triple-blind:* In addition to participants and researchers, the analysts who interpret the data are also kept unaware of the group assignments, further minimizing bias.

Blinding is a critical component in ensuring the integrity and reliability of research findings.

Epidemiology

Epidemiology is the branch of medical science that studies the distribution, determinants, and deterrents of health-related states and events in specified populations. It plays a crucial role in public health by identifying risk factors for disease and targets for preventive healthcare. Epidemiologists work on studying the patterns, causes, and effects of health and disease conditions in defined populations, providing the foundation for interventions and policy development aimed at improving public health outcomes.

Epidemiological Methods

The primary concern of the epidemiologist is to study disease occurrence in people who, during the course of their lives, are exposed to numerous factors and circumstances, some of which may have a role in disease etiology. Unlike the clinician or the laboratory investigator, who is above to study disease conditions more precisely, the epidemiologist employs carefully designed research strategies to explore disease etiology.

Epidemiological studies can be classified as observational studies and experimental studies with further subdivisions **(Table 1.5)**.

TABLE 1.5: Classification of epidemiological studies.

Observational studies	Experimental studies
Descriptive studies	Experimental or interventional studies
Analytical studies	Randomized or nonrandomized clinical trials
Ecological or correlational	Field trials
Cross-sectional or prevalence	Community trials
Case control	
Cohort	

"Retrospective" Studies in the Clinical Setting versus Population Setting

Studies where data are retrieved from case records or electronic medical records (EMR) and analyzed for various observations are also typically referred to as *retrospective studies*. In a retrospective study, researchers analyze existing data to find correlations, outcomes, and trends. This type of study involves reviewing historical records and data sets that were collected for other purposes, rather than conducting new experiments or surveys.

Retrospective studies are often used in fields, such as medicine, epidemiology, and social sciences to identify patterns, risk factors, and long-term effects. By examining large amounts of past data, researchers can generate hypotheses and inform future research directions, although they must be careful to account for potential biases and limitations inherent in the original data sources.

To distinguish "retrospective" studies conducted in clinical environments from those performed in population settings, it is essential for studies categorized under retrospective studies to take into account the following considerations:

- *Data source:* Retrospective studies using EMR data focus on healthcare records collected during routine patient care, while epidemiological studies might use a broader range of data sources, including surveys, disease registries, and public health records.
- *Scope and purpose:* EMR-based retrospective studies often aim to evaluate clinical outcomes, treatment efficacy, or patient characteristics in a specific healthcare setting. Epidemiological studies, on the other hand, generally aim to study the distribution and determinants of health-related states or events in a population.
- *Type of analysis:* While both study types can use similar analytical methods, epidemiological studies might focus more on the prevalence, incidence, and risk factors of diseases within a population, whereas EMR-based studies might prioritize clinical outcomes and patient care quality.

■ STUDY DESIGNS

Based on exposure study designs have been classified into two major subtypes—observational studies or experimental or interventional studies.

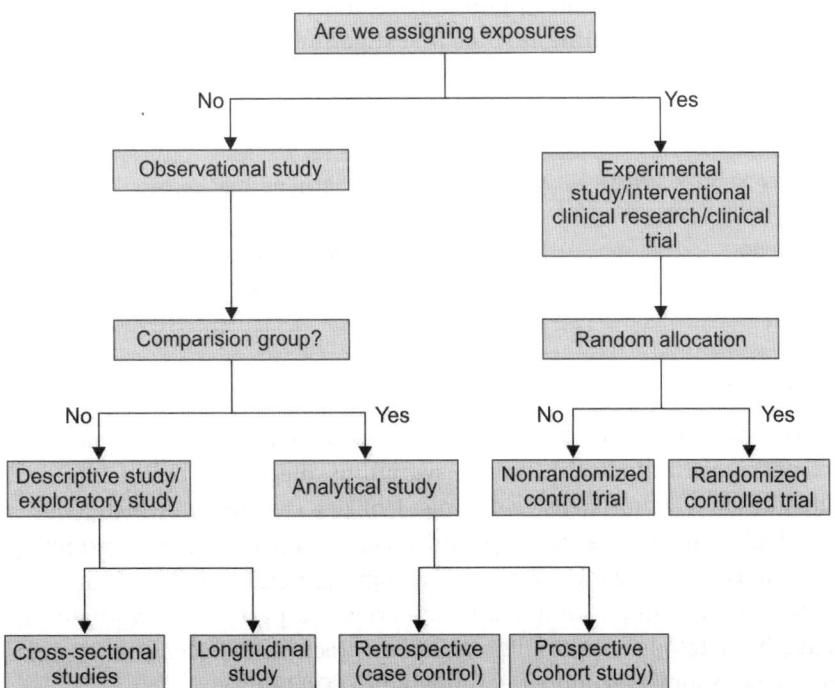

Flowchart 1.1: Flowchart representing study designs from the field of epidemiology and clinical research.

Observational Studies

As the name suggests, this type of study involves only observations without any intervention, such as treatment and surgery, being administered to the study subjects. For example, if we aim to identify an association between cigarette smoking and glaucoma among the Indian population.

In the example above, cigarette smoking is considered a habit or addiction, while glaucoma is classified as a disease. The investigator will observe any correlation between smoking and glaucoma without introducing any intervention. Therefore, this constitutes an observational study.

Subtypes of observational studies:
- Case reports
- Case series
- Descriptive studies
- Analytical Studies

Case Report

A case report is a detailed presentation of a single patient's medical history, symptoms, diagnosis, treatment, and follow-up. It often highlights a rare or novel condition, treatment, or outcome, providing valuable clinical insights and contributing to medical knowledge. Case reports can serve as the first line of evidence in identifying new diseases or adverse effects of treatments, prompting further investigation through more extensive studies **(Table 1.6)**.

TABLE 1.6: Case report of a single patient presenting with a rare disease.	
Case report of "Four years follow-up of stable ultrathin nonectatic cornea: A case report"	
Case report	Only one patient was followed up for four years to see the progression of changes in corneal keratometry readings and curvature over four years

Case Series

A case series involves a group of patients with a similar diagnosis or treatment, presenting their medical histories, symptoms, diagnoses, treatments, and outcomes in a comprehensive manner. Unlike a case report, which focuses on a single patient, a case series provides a broader perspective by examining multiple cases, allowing for pattern recognition and the identification of commonalities and variations. Case series are particularly valuable in highlighting trends, rare conditions, or new treatment effects, and they can pave the way for larger, more rigorous studies **(Table 1.7)**.

TABLE 1.7: Case series involving 16 patients.	
Case series: "Corneal collagen crosslinking for the treatment of microbial keratitis"	
Case series	Here in the above case series, 16 patients were included and underwent corneal collagen cross-linking for treatment of microbial keratitis. 16 patients were only included, which is why it is a case series

Case reports and series are considered prestudy ventures, i.e., strictly speaking, they are not studies; they are preliminary research investigations studying single or very few subjects.

Descriptive Studies

The best study of mankind is man. This statement emphasizes the importance of making the best use of observations on individuals or populations exposed to suspected factors of disease. Meticulous observations made in Africa by Burkitt led to the eventual incrimination of Epstein–Barr virus (EBV) as the etiological factor (possibly conditioned by other factors such as malaria infection) of the type of cancer known as Burkitt's lymphoma.

Descriptive studies are usually the first phase of an epidemiological investigation. These studies are concerned with observing the distribution of disease or health-related characteristics in human populations and identifying the characteristics with which the disease in question seems to be associated. Such studies basically ask questions.

Basic steps or procedures in descriptive studies:
- *Defining the population to be studied:* Defining the population to be studied is a critical step in any descriptive study. This involves selecting a group of individuals who share common characteristics relevant to the research question. The population could be defined by geographic location, age, gender, ethnicity, occupation, or any other pertinent demographic factor. The clarity in defining the population ensures that the findings are specific, reliable, and can potentially be generalized to a larger group.
- *Defining the disease under study:* Once the population has been defined, the next step is to clearly define the disease or health-related outcome being studied. This entails establishing precise diagnostic criteria and case definitions to accurately identify cases within the population. These definitions should be as specific and consistent as possible to ensure that all cases are identified accurately and there is no misclassification.
- *Describing the disease by time, place, and person:* Descriptive studies often categorize disease occurrences by time, place, and person to identify patterns and trends.

- *Time:* This involves examining when the disease occurs, considering factors, such as the season, year, and specific events. Temporal patterns can reveal outbreaks, seasonal trends, or long-term changes in disease rates. For example, an increase in respiratory diseases during winter could indicate the influence of colder weather on disease prevalence.
- *Place:* Place analysis focuses on the geographic locations where the disease occurs. It helps in identifying areas with higher or lower disease rates, which may be due to environmental factors, population density, or access to healthcare services. Maps and spatial analysis tools can visually represent these geographic patterns, aiding in pinpointing hotspots or regions at risk.
- *Person:* Examining person characteristics involves analyzing who is affected by the disease, considering variables such as age, gender, ethnicity, occupation, and socioeconomic status. This helps in identifying vulnerable groups and understanding the demographic distribution of the disease. For example, certain diseases may disproportionately affect children, the elderly, or specific ethnic groups.

  By systematically describing the disease in terms of time, place, and person, researchers can generate hypotheses about potential causes, identify risk factors, and develop targeted interventions to control and prevent the disease.
- *Measurement of disease:* It is mandatory to have a clear picture of the amount of disease in the population. This information should be available in terms of mortality, morbidity, disability, and so on, and should preferably be available for different subgroups of the population. Incidence and prevalence being two important aspects of disease; incidence can be obtained from longitudinal studies, and prevalence from cross-sectional studies.

Cross-sectional studies: Cross-sectional studies are observational studies that analyze data from a population, or a representative subset, at a specific point in time. These studies are particularly useful for assessing the prevalence of a disease or health-related outcome within the population. By collecting data at a single point in time, researchers can determine how widespread a condition is and identify potential associations between the disease and various demographic or environmental factors **(Flowchart 1.2)** **(Table 1.8)**.

One of the advantages of cross-sectional studies is their efficiency in terms of time and resources, as they provide a snapshot of the population's health status without the need for long-term follow-up. They are also valuable for hypothesis generation, as they can highlight trends and correlations that

Flowchart 1.2: Cross-sectional study design.

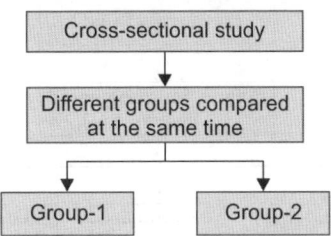

TABLE 1.8: Cross-sectional studies represented in an article.	
Cross-sectional studies: "Assessment of awareness of keratoconus and its relation to eye rubbing among the Saudi Arabian population"	
Cross-sectional study	• A quantitative survey was conducted from March 2024 to July 2024 over a period of 4 months in Saudi Arabia to assess the level of awareness regarding keratoconus (KC) and its relation to eye rubbing among residents from various regions of Saudi Arabia • Participants were randomly selected, and questionnaires were distributed via self-administered Google Forms. The sample size was 2,059 participants to address potential issues with missing data or incomplete forms • Here, as each patient filled in the form once, i.e., was surveyed at one point of time, only this is a cross-sectional study

warrant further investigation through more rigorous study designs. However, cross-sectional studies have limitations, including the inability to establish causality due to the simultaneous measurement of exposure and outcome.

Longitudinal studies: Longitudinal studies are observational studies that involve repeated observations of the same variables over extended periods of time, often years or even decades. These studies are pivotal in understanding the incidence and natural history of diseases, as they track the development and progression of health outcomes within a cohort **(Flowchart 1.3)**.

By following the same group of individuals, longitudinal studies can capture changes in health status and identify potential causal relationships between exposures and outcomes. This design allows researchers to distinguish between incidence (new cases of disease) and prevalence (existing cases of disease), providing valuable insights into the dynamics of disease occurrence.

One of the main advantages of longitudinal studies is their ability to establish temporal sequences, thereby strengthening the evidence for causal inferences. Additionally, longitudinal studies can identify latent periods,

Flowchart 1.3: Longitudinal study.

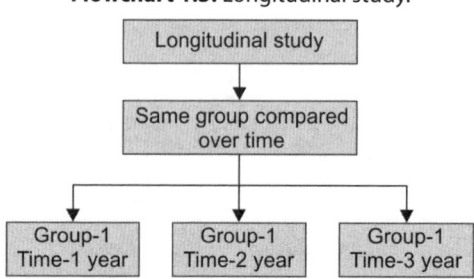

TABLE 1.9: Longitudinal study to assess retinal and choroidal changes in divers.	
Longitudinal study: "Retinal layer and choroidal changes in deep and scuba divers: Evidence of pachychoroid spectrum-like findings"	
Longitudinal study	• The study is to evaluate the long-term effects of diving on the thicknesses of retinal layers and retinal anatomy in professional deep and scuba divers. The study included 52 eyes of deep divers, 49 scuba divers, and 66 eyes of the control group. Measurements of macular retinal layer thicknesses, peripapillary nerve fiber layer thickness, and subfoveal choroidal thickness were performed and statistically compared between the groups. The retinal pigment epithelium (RPE) and subfoveal choroidal thickness were statistically significantly thicker in deep divers than in the scuba divers and control group. An increased thickening of the subfoveal choroid and RPE, resembling pachychoroid pigment epitheliopathy, was detected in deep divers over a long-term duration • As the study involved long-term follow-up without any intervention (diving being a lifestyle choice), this is an example of a longitudinal study

during which the effects of an exposure may not be immediately apparent but manifest later.

However, longitudinal studies also have challenges, including the need for substantial time and resources to maintain follow-up with participants. Attrition, or loss of participants over time, can introduce bias and affect the study's validity. Despite these limitations, longitudinal studies remain a cornerstone of epidemiological research, providing critical data for understanding disease etiology and informing public health interventions **(Table 1.9)**.

- *Comparing with known indices:* By making comparisons between different populations and subgroups of the same population, it is possible to arrive at clues to disease etiology.
- *Formulation of an etiological hypothesis:* By studying the distribution of disease, and utilizing he techniques of descriptive epidemiology, it is

often possible to formulate hypotheses relating to disease etiology. By observing attributes of a population, it is possible to formulate hypotheses or suppositions about the causal etiology of a disease.

Analytical Studies

Analytical studies are designed to test specific hypotheses regarding the relationships between exposures and outcomes. These studies are crucial in establishing causality and identifying risk factors for diseases. In contrast to descriptive studies, where the entire population is studied, in an analytical study the subject of interest is the individual within the population. The object is not to formulate. But to test hypotheses.

There are several types of analytical studies, each with its unique methodology and applications.
- Ecological studies
- Case-control study
- Cohort study

Ecological studies: Ecological or correlational studies examine the relationships between exposure and health outcomes on a population level rather than an individual level. These studies often utilize existing data, such as national health statistics, to identify patterns and correlations that may warrant further investigation.

Case-control studies: Case-control studies compare individuals with a specific disease (cases) to those without the disease (controls) to identify factors that may contribute to the disease's development.

Case-control studies are retrospective in nature, meaning they look back in time to compare the history of exposure in cases and controls. These studies are efficient for investigating diseases with long latency periods, as they can quickly gather data without waiting for a disease to develop in a study population.

One of the key strengths of case-control studies is their ability to study rare diseases. Since these studies focus on individuals who already have the disease, they do not require a large sample size to identify significant associations. Researchers can also investigate multiple exposures for a single outcome, providing valuable insights into potential risk factors **(Flowchart 1.4)**.

However, case-control studies also have limitations. The reliance on historical data can lead to recall bias, where individuals may not accurately remember their past exposures. Additionally, selecting appropriate control groups can be challenging, as they must be similar to cases in every aspect except for the presence of the disease **(Table 1.10)**.

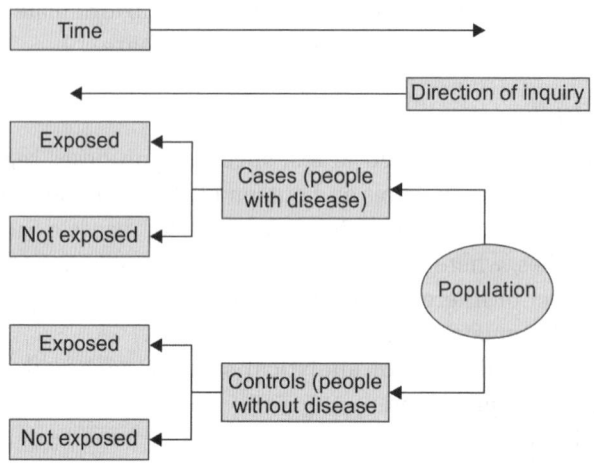

Flowchart 1.4: Flowchart representing a case-control study.

TABLE 1.10: Example of a case-control study.	
Case-control study "The effect of cigarette smoking on corneal endothelial cells"	
Case-control study	• The study included 99 participants, 61 chronic cigarette smokers (Cases) and another age matched 38 (control) nonsmokers. Various endothelial cell parameters were compared between the cases and controls, like cell density (CD), polymegethism, pleomorphism, the average of cell size, and central corneal thickness (CCT). A statistically significant change in endothelial parameters among the cases as compared to the control was noted • *Conclusion:* Cigarette smoking has deteriorating effects on corneal endothelial measures. As the study compared cases and controls, i.e., smokers and nonsmokers, this is a case-control study

Despite these challenges, case-control studies remain a fundamental tool in epidemiological research. They have contributed to significant findings in public health, such as the link between smoking and lung cancer, and continue to be instrumental in identifying risk factors for various diseases.

Cohort studies: Cohort studies follow a group of individuals over time to assess the impact of different exposures on the development of specific health outcomes. These studies can be prospective, following participants into the future, or retrospective, using historical data to reconstruct exposure histories. Cohort studies are powerful tools for identifying risk factors and establishing temporal relationships between exposures and outcomes. **(Flowchart 1.5) (Table 1.11)**.

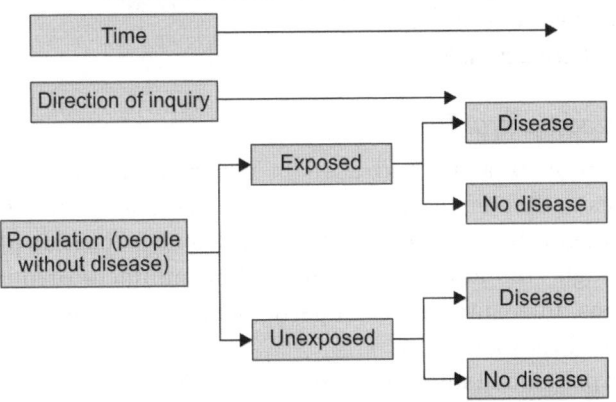

Flowchart 1.5: Flowchart of cohort study.

TABLE 1.11: Representing a cohort study of a group of patients undergoing phacoemulsification.	
Cohort study: "Unhappy patients after uneventful phacoemulsification"	
Cohort study	To assess the prevalence and causes of unhappy patients after uneventful phacoemulsification: *The study included* 100 patients who underwent uncomplicated phacoemulsification in the period from February to April 2024 with the same surgeon. Patients were followed up after 2 months of surgery. All selected patients were recalled and subjected to a face-to-face questionnaire to measure their satisfaction level. In the dissatisfied group, all patients were subjected to full history taking, visual acuity assessment, anterior and posterior segment examinations, ultrasonography, and optical coherence tomography. As the study included the same group of patients (cohort and assessed their outcome over a period of time, whether satisfied or dissatisfied) this is an example of a cohort study

Experimental/Interventional Study

Experimental or interventional studies are designed to test hypotheses by manipulating one or more variables and observing the effects on specific outcomes. Unlike observational studies, which merely observe and analyze existing data, experimental studies involve actively intervening, i.e., by administration of therapeutics either as drugs or surgeries, and controlling conditions to establish causal relationships. Randomization plays a crucial role in experimental studies (randomization has already been described in **Chapter 4** on Sampling Techniques). After selection of the study population, they are randomized into two or more groups to eliminate selection bias and balance confounding variables across groups, thus ensuring that any observed differences in outcomes can be attributed to the intervention rather than other factors.

Based on randomization, it can be classified into two types:
1. Randomized control trials
2. Nonrandomized trials

Randomized Control Trials

Randomization is a method used in experimental studies to assign participants to different groups, such as treatment or control groups, in an unbiased manner. This process involves randomly allocating participants, often through computer-generated random numbers or other chance mechanisms, to ensure that each participant has an equal probability of being placed in any given group.

In an experimental study, participants are assigned to either the treatment group, which receives the intervention, or the control group, which does not. This randomization helps to eliminate bias and ensures that any differences observed between the groups can be attributed to the intervention itself rather than other factors. The most rigorous form of experimental study is the RCT, often considered the gold standard in clinical research.

Randomized controlled trials are commonly used to evaluate the efficacy and safety of new medical treatments, drugs, or interventions. By comparing outcomes between the treatment and control groups, researchers can determine whether the intervention significantly impacts health outcomes. For example, an RCT might be conducted to assess the effectiveness of a new vaccine in preventing a disease.

One of the advantages of experimental studies is their ability to establish cause-and-effect relationships with a high degree of confidence. By controlling for confounding variables and using randomization, researchers can isolate the effect of the intervention and make strong inferences about its impact.

However, experimental studies also have limitations. They can be expensive and time-consuming to conduct, requiring significant resources and careful planning. Additionally, ethical considerations may arise when withholding potentially beneficial treatments from control groups or exposing participants to potential risks. Despite these challenges, experimental studies remain a critical component of scientific research, providing invaluable insights into the effectiveness and safety of interventions across various fields **(Table 1.12)**.

Nonrandomized Trials

Nonrandomized control trials, on the other hand, do not involve the random assignment of participants to treatment and control groups. Instead, participants are allocated to groups based on predetermined criteria or

TABLE 1.12: Illustration for the randomized control study.

Comparing adjuvant beta radiation, mitomycin C, and conjunctival autograft in primary pterygium treatment, a 3-year follow-up study

Randomized controlled trial	The study included 180 eyes undergoing primary pterygium excision followed by adjuvant therapy using Beta radiation, mitomycin C (0.02% for 5 minutes), or conjunctival autograft. The patients were randomly divided into three groups, each comprising 60 patients. Group (A) received Beta radiation following pterygium excision, group (B) had primary pterygium excision with the application of 0.02% mitomycin C for 5 minutes, and group (C) had a conjunctival autograft to cover the bare area after pterygium excision. Patients were followed up for 3 years postoperatively. Group A had a recurrence rate of 33.3%, group B had a recurrence rate of 13.3%, and group C had a recurrence rate of 6.7%. Group B showed the highest rate of intraocular postoperative complications, while no intraocular complications were recorded in group C. Common complications in groups A and B included scleral melting, keratitis, and Dellen formation. The use of conjunctival autograft after primary pterygium excision resulted in the lowest rate of recurrence and postoperative complications. In contrast, Beta radiation or Mitomycin C did not show as favorable results. As patients were randomized into three groups based on a computer-generated sequence, it is a randomized study

natural occurrences, which can introduce bias and affect the internal validity of the study. While nonrandomized trials can provide valuable information, their ability to establish causal relationships is generally weaker compared to RCTs **(Table 1.13)**.

In nonrandomized trials, researchers must employ additional statistical techniques, and careful study designs to account for potential confounding variables and biases. These studies are often used when randomization is impractical or unethical. For example, nonrandomized trials might be employed in public health research where interventions are implemented at the community level and randomization is not feasible.

Despite their limitations, nonrandomized control trials can still offer significant insights, particularly in real-world settings where strict control and randomization are not possible. They can help identify trends, generate hypotheses, and provide preliminary evidence on the effectiveness of interventions. Ultimately, nonrandomized control trials complement RCTs, contributing to a more comprehensive understanding of various interventions and their impacts.

TABLE 1.13: Nonrandomized clinical trial.

Nonrandomized study: "Optical coherence tomography angiography after ranibizumab treatment for diabetic macular edema.

Nonrandomized trial	The study assessed changes and ischemia that may occur post. Injection using OCT and OCTA and its relationship with BCVA. A total of 49 eyes were enrolled in the study to evaluate changes in central macular thickness, visual acuity, foveal avascular zone, and vascular density following intravitreal injection of ranibizumab used in patients diagnosed with central involving diabetic macular edema. As all patients were included, no randomization was done

(BCVA: best corrected visual acuity; OCT: optical coherence tomography; OCTA: optical coherence tomography angiography)

ADVANCED STUDY DESIGNS

- Systematic reviews
- Meta-analysis

Systematic Reviews

Systematic reviews are a rigorous and methodical approach to synthesizing research evidence on a specific topic. By identifying, evaluating, and integrating the findings from multiple studies, systematic reviews aim to provide a comprehensive and unbiased summary of the available evidence. This process involves several key steps:

- *Formulating a research question:* The first step is to define a clear and focused research question that guides the review process. This question typically follows the PICO framework, which stands for population, intervention, comparison, and outcomes.
- *Developing a protocol:* A detailed protocol outlines the methods and criteria for the systematic review. This protocol is often registered in databases such as PROSPERO to enhance transparency and reduce potential bias.
- *Conducting a comprehensive literature search:* Researchers perform an exhaustive search of relevant databases, journals, and other sources to identify all studies that meet the inclusion criteria. This search is designed to capture both published and unpublished research to avoid publication bias.
- *Screening and selecting studies:* The identified studies are screened for eligibility based on predefined inclusion and exclusion criteria. This step ensures that only studies relevant to the research question are included in the review.

- *Assessing the quality of studies:* Each selected study is critically appraised for methodological quality and risk of bias. Tools such as the Cochrane Risk of Bias tool are commonly used for this purpose.
- *Extracting and analyzing data:* Data from the studies included are systematically extracted and analyzed. This may involve both qualitative and quantitative synthesis methods, depending on the nature of the data.
- *Interpreting and reporting findings:* The results of the systematic review are interpreted in the context of the overall body of evidence. Researchers consider the strength, consistency, and applicability of the findings and report them in a transparent and structured manner.

Systematic reviews are invaluable in evidence-based practice, as they aggregate and distill a vast amount of research into actionable insights. By providing a high level of evidence, they inform clinical guidelines, policy decisions, and future research directions, ultimately contributing to improved outcomes in various fields.

Meta-analysis

Meta-analysis is a statistical technique that combines results from multiple studies on the same topic. This method improves the accuracy of effect size estimates and enhances the power to find significant effects. Key steps include **(Table 1.14)**:

- *Formulating research questions and hypotheses:* Begin with a clear research question and hypotheses to guide study selection and analysis.
- *Literature search and study selection:* Conduct a thorough search for relevant studies, selecting those that meet predefined criteria.
- *Data extraction:* Extract key data like sample size and effect size for quantitative analysis.
- *Assessing study quality and risk of bias:* Evaluate each study's quality and potential bias using standardized tools.

TABLE 1.14: Illustration for the meta analysis.	
Meta-analysis: "Lifitegrast in treatment of dry eye disease—a practical, narrative expert review"	
Meta-analysis	The above study included 14 published studies collected from the PubMed database to analyze the data and demonstrate the role of lifitegrast, an immunomodulator in dry eyes. The aim of the review was to critically evaluate the literature already published from multiple sources concerning the efficacy and safety of lifitegrast, a small molecule immunomodulator that blocks the action of lymphocyte function-associated antigen-1. The study found that it had a positive role in reducing the incidence of dry eyes

- *Statistical analysis*: Use statistical methods to calculate the combined effect size, considering variability among studies.
- *Heterogeneity assessment*: Measure variability among studies with tests like the I^2 statistic.
- *Publication bias assessment*: Check for publication bias using funnel plots and Egger's test.
- *Interpreting and reporting results*: Interpret results in the context of overall evidence, considering effect size, consistency, and biases, then report findings transparently.
- Meta-analysis strengthens research findings by synthesizing multiple studies, informing clinical practice, policy-making, and future research.

■ CONCLUSION

In conclusion, the design of studies plays a critical role in ensuring the reliability and validity of research findings. Properly designed studies facilitate accurate statistical analysis, robust assessment of heterogeneity. By adhering to rigorous methodological standards, researchers can produce high-quality evidence that contributes to the body of knowledge, informs clinical practice, guides policymaking, and lays the groundwork for future investigations. Meticulous design and transparent reporting of studies are fundamental to the advancement of science and the credibility of research outcomes.

■ SUGGESTED READING

1. Ali S, Elagouz M, Sayed Kh, Abdellah M. Optical coherence tomography angiography after ranibizumab treatment for diabetic macular edema. Egypt J Clin Ophthalmol [Internet]. 2023 (cited 2023/06/01);6(1):75-83. Available from: https://doi.org/10.21608/ejco.2023.305207
2. Alqasimi NA, Aljohani LH, Ambrósio R, AlQahtani BS, Al Haydar NS, Alanazi, BR, et al. Frontiers | Assessment of awareness of keratoconus and its relation to eye rubbing among Saudi Arabia population. Front Ophthalmol [Internet]. 2025 (cited 2025/02/11);5. Available from: https://doi.org/10.3389/fopht.2025.1545030
3. Al-Salem KM, Saif ATS, Saif PS. Comparing Adjuvant Beta Radiation, Mitomycin C, and Conjunctival Autograft in Primary Pterygium Treatment, a Three-year Follow-up Study. Open Ophthalmol J [Internet]. 2020 (cited 2020/12/31);14(1). Available from: https://doi.org/10.2174/1874364102014010082
4. Demir N, Kayhan B, Acar M, Sevincli S, Sonmez M. Retinal Layer and Choroidal Changes in Deep and Scuba Divers: Evidence of Pachychoroid Spectrum-Like Findings. J Ophthalmol [Internet]. 2024 (cited 2024/01/01);2024(1). Available from: https://doi.org/10.1155/2024/1600148
5. El Saman I, Mohamed O, Kamel A. The effect of cigarette smoking on corneal endothelial cells. Egypt J Clin Ophthalmol [Internet]. 2019

(cited 2019/06/01);2(1):5-11. Available from: https://doi.org/10.21608/ejco.2019.162995

6. Hamza A, Abd El-Rahman M, Ali T, El-Sebaity D. Corneal collagen crosslinking for the treatment of microbial keratitis. Egypt J Clin Ophthalmol [Internet]. 2022 (cited 2022/12/01);5(2):67-77. Available from: https://doi.org/10.21608/ejco.2022.280969

7. He M, Wang W, Zhang X, Huang W. Ologen implant versus mitomycin C for trabeculectomy: a systematic review and meta-analysis. PLoS One [Internet]. 2014 (cited 20/01/2014);9(1):e85782. Available from: https://doi.org/10.1371/journal.pone.0085782

8. Herrinton LJ, Liu L, Alexeeff S, Carolan J, Shorstein NH. Immediate Sequential vs. Delayed Sequential Bilateral Cataract Surgery: Retrospective Comparison of Postoperative Visual Outcomes. Ophthalmology [Internet]. 2017(cited 2017);124(8):1126-35. Available from: https://doi.org/10.1016/j.ophtha.2017.03.034

9. Landsend ECS, Istre M, Utheim TP. Lifitegrast in treatment of dry eye disease—a practical, narrative expert review. J Ophthalmol [Internet]. 2025 (cited 2025/01/01);2025(1). Available from: https://doi.org/10.1155/joph/6504111

10. Mohammed M. Unhappy patients after uneventful phacoemulsification. Egypt J Clin Ophthalmol [Internet]. 2024 (cited 2024/12/01);7(2):147-57. Available from: https://doi.org/10.21608/ejco.2024.404125

11. Nagy Kh, Elshorbagy S, El Hariry A, Mounir A. Four years follow up of stable ultrathin non ectatic cornea: a case report. Egypt J Clin Ophthalmol [Internet]. 2022 (cited 2022/12/01);5(2):61-65. Available from: https://doi.org/10.21608/ejco.2022.280968

12. Yousef H, Gad Elkareem A, El Rawy E. Correlation between visual acuity and outer retinal layer thickness in diabetic macular edema. Egypt J Clin Ophthalmol [Internet]. 2024 (cited 2024/12/01);7(2). Available from: https://doi.org/10.21608/ejco.2024.404121

13. Yuan Y, Xiong R, Wu Y, Ha J, Wang W, Han X et al. Associations of statin use with the onset and progression of open-angle glaucoma: A systematic review and meta-analysis. EClinicalMedicine [Internet]. 2022 (cited 2022);46:101364. Available from: https://doi.org/10.1016/j.eclinm.2022.101364

APPENDIX 2

Research Project Flow: From Idea to Innovation

Sunil Moreker, Ditsha Datta

■ INTRODUCTION

In the realm of medical research, the journey from conceptualization to innovation is one of profound transformation and meticulous execution. This chapter delves into the fascinating expedition that begins with a spark of curiosity and culminates in advancements that push the boundaries of medical knowledge and practice. It explores the systematic flow of a research project, illustrating how an initial idea, often born from pressing clinical dilemmas, evolves through rigorous phases of hypothesis formulation, ethical scrutiny, and comprehensive study design. This odyssey, undertaken by dedicated clinicians and researchers, embodies the relentless quest for scientific truth and the commitment to enhancing patient care. By navigating the intricate pathways of research and publication, this chapter aims to illuminate the processes that underpin groundbreaking discoveries and underscore the significance of each step in the journey toward medical innovation.

■ FROM CLINICAL DILEMMA TO PUBLICATION: THE EVOLUTION OF AN IDEA

The journey from an initial clinical dilemma to a published research paper in ophthalmology is a multifaceted process that transforms an idea into a significant contribution to medical knowledge. This pathway encompasses several critical steps, including the genesis of the research hypothesis, addressing ethical considerations, meticulous study design, and the actual conduct of the study.

A Journey Through the Research and Publishing Process

This intricate voyage, often embarked upon by passionate and inquisitive clinicians, weaves through the labyrinthine corridors of scientific inquiry. It is a testament to the relentless pursuit of knowledge and the commitment to advancing ophthalmic care. Each stage of this journey builds upon the last, with the ultimate aim of shedding light on previously uncharted territories and enhancing patient outcomes.

The Genesis of an Idea

Every ophthalmology study begins with a clinical dilemma encountered by a clinician. This initial problem can arise from a challenging case, a recurring issue in patient care, or an unexplored area in ophthalmology. The clinician's expertise and curiosity drive them to seek answers and solutions, laying the groundwork for a potential research study.

Formulating a Hypothesis

In scientific research, formulating a hypothesis is a crucial step. A hypothesis is a testable statement that predicts an outcome based on certain variables. For an ophthalmology study, this might involve predicting the effectiveness of a new treatment, the cause of a particular condition, or the impact of a diagnostic method. This hypothesis drives the direction of the research and helps to focus the study on specific objectives.

Ethical Considerations

Before proceeding with the study, ethical considerations must be addressed. This involves ensuring that the research adheres to ethical guidelines and protects the rights and well-being of participants. Clinicians must obtain approval from an institutional review board (IRB) or ethics committee, which reviews the study's design, consent process, and potential risks. Ethical approval is essential for maintaining the integrity of the research and safeguarding participants.

Study Design

Once the hypothesis is formulated and ethical approval is obtained, the next step is designing the study. This includes selecting the appropriate methodology, choosing the sample size, and determining the tools for data collection. In ophthalmology, study designs may range from clinical trials and cohort studies to case-control studies and observational research. The study design ensures that the research is systematic and replicable, providing reliable results that contribute to the field of ophthalmology.

Conduct of the Study

With the study design in place, the actual research begins. This phase involves recruiting participants, collecting data, and meticulously documenting findings. Clinicians and researchers must adhere to the study protocol, ensuring that the data is accurate and unbiased. In ophthalmology, this might include conducting eye examinations, administering treatments, and monitoring patient outcomes over time.

Data Analysis

After data collection is complete, the next step is analyzing the data. This involves using statistical methods to interpret the results and determine whether the hypothesis is supported. Data analysis helps identify patterns, correlations, and significant findings that can advance understanding in ophthalmology. Researchers may use software tools and collaborate with biostatisticians to ensure robust and accurate analysis.

Manuscript Preparation

With the results analyzed, the clinician can begin preparing the manuscript. This involves writing a detailed report of the study, including the background, methodology, results, and conclusions. The manuscript should be clear, concise, and well-organized, providing valuable insights to the ophthalmology community. Authors may seek feedback from colleagues and mentors to refine the manuscript before submission.

Submission and Peer Review

Once the manuscript is polished, it is submitted to a reputable medical journal for publication. The journal's editorial team conducts an initial review, followed by a peer-review process where experts in the field evaluate the study's quality, validity, and contribution to ophthalmology. Peer review is a critical step that ensures the research meets high standards and provides reliable information to readers.

Publication, Patent, and Application

If the manuscript passes peer review, it is accepted for publication and becomes part of the scientific literature. The published study can influence clinical practice, guide future research, and contribute to the ongoing advancement of ophthalmology.

In some cases, research may lead to a patent, particularly if it involves a new treatment, device, or diagnostic method. Securing a patent protects intellectual property and allows for commercialization, further extending the impact of the research.

Dissemination and Impact

Following publication or patent, the research findings are disseminated to the wider medical community. This can involve presenting at conferences, sharing through professional networks, and engaging with media outlets. Effective dissemination ensures that the knowledge reaches clinicians, researchers, and policymakers, ultimately improving patient care and advancing the field of ophthalmology.

Legacy and Future Research

The journey from clinical dilemma to publication or patent is a testament to the dedication, creativity, and perseverance of the clinician-researcher.

The findings contribute to the collective knowledge of ophthalmology and can inspire future research projects. The legacy of the research lies in its potential to improve patient outcomes, inform clinical practice, and drive innovation in the field. Ultimately, the process exemplifies the continuous quest for knowledge and the pursuit of excellence in ophthalmology.

DIFFERENCES IN THE JOURNEY OF A BEGINNER RESIDENT VERSUS A SEASONED CLINICIAN (TABLE 2.1)

The journey from clinical inquiry to impactful research in ophthalmology is a multifaceted process that demands rigorous effort and unwavering dedication. This exploration begins with identifying a clinical dilemma, followed by a methodical investigation designed to uncover novel insights or validate existing practices. Such endeavors are crucial for advancing the field,

TABLE 2.1: The journey of research for the beginner versus the seasoned clinician.

Aspect	Beginner resident	Seasoned clinician
Approach to Ideas	Primarily focused on learning and understanding existing knowledge. May generate ideas based on observed gaps or questions during training	More likely to generate novel ideas based on extensive experience and a deep understanding of the field. Identifies innovative solutions to complex problems
Mentorship and collaboration	Relies heavily on guidance from mentors and collaborating with peers to refine ideas. Limited autonomy in pursuing independent research	Often serves as a mentor and collaborates with other experts. Has greater autonomy and resources to pursue innovative research projects
Resources and support	Access to limited resources and support is primarily within the training program. Innovations are often small-scale and supervised	Access to extensive resources, funding, and institutional support. Capable of leading large-scale research projects and clinical trials
Impact of innovations	Innovations may have a localized impact within the training environment or a specific department. Focus on learning and incremental improvements	Innovations can have a significant impact on clinical practice, patient care, and the broader field. Focus on transformative changes and advancements
Risk and experimentation	Limited capacity for taking risks due to the need for supervision and adherence to established protocols	Greater willingness and ability to take calculated risks and experiment with new approaches. Can challenge conventional practices with evidence-based innovations

improving patient care, and fostering innovation. This overview highlights the key stages of this journey, from manuscript submission and peer review to publication, patenting, and dissemination, illustrating the profound impact research can have on the medical community and beyond.

For a beginner resident, this journey is often characterized by a heavy reliance on mentorship and collaboration, with a focus on learning and understanding existing knowledge. They may generate ideas based on observed gaps or questions during their training. In contrast, a seasoned clinician is more likely to generate novel ideas based on extensive experience and a deep understanding of the field. They often serve as mentors themselves and have greater autonomy and resources to pursue innovative research projects, identifying innovative solutions to complex problems.

■ CONCLUSION

The transition from a training environment to a fully supported professional setting marks a pivotal evolution in the capacity for innovation within the field. While the foundational stage fosters incremental learning and cautious experimentation, the advanced stage leverages extensive resources and institutional backing to drive significant advancements and transformative changes.

This progression not only enhances clinical practices and patient care but also propels the broader field toward a future replete with evidence-based innovations that challenge and refine conventional methodologies.

■ SUGGESTED READING

1. Articles: "Disruptive Innovation for Social Change" by Clayton M. Christensen, Heiner Baumann, Rudy Ruggles, and Thomas M. Sadtler (Harvard Business Review)
2. Crossing the Chasm: Marketing and Selling High-Tech Products to Mainstream Customers by Geoffrey A. Moore
3. Innovation and Entrepreneurship by Peter F. Drucker
4. "Lean Healthcare: Innovation in Hospitals" by Toussaint and Gerard (Healthcare Quarterly)
5. The Innovator's Prescription: A Disruptive Solution for Health Care by Clayton M. Christensen, Jerome H. Grossman, and Jason Hwang
6. The Innovator's Dilemma: When New Technologies Cause Great Firms to Fail by Clayton M. Christensen
7. The Lean Startup: How Today's Entrepreneurs Use Continuous Innovation to Create Radically Successful Businesses by Eric Ries
8. "The Role of Incremental and Radical Innovation in the Development of New Product Offerings" by Abbie Griffin, John Hauser, and Steven Urban (Journal of Marketing Research)

Index

Page numbers followed by *b* refer to box, *f* refer to figure, *fc* refer to flowchart, and *t* refer to table.

A

Accuracy, degree of 153
Advanced statistical
    methods 170
    modeling 166
    techniques 17
Advanced study designs 208
Age-related eye condition 89
Alternative hypothesis 107, 108, 118-119, 122, 126, 127
    one-sided 108
    two-sided 108
Analysis of variance 75, 86, 112, 121, 123, 124, 126-129, 134, 136, 137, 147, 150, 163
    application, content for 124t
    concept of 123t
    repeated measures 153t
    test 128t, 129t
    types of 122
Analysis
    results, clear presentation of 190
    type of 197
Analytical methods, robustness of 8
Analytical studies 198, 203
Analyzing data 209
Analyzing diagnostic reliability sensitivity and specificity 138t
Angiotensin-converting enzyme 123
Angle opening distance 131
Anomalies, discussion of 190
Anonymization protocols 189
Anterior chamber depth 24
Arithmetic mean
    classification of 54f
    demerits of 57
    merits of 57
    properties of 55
Artificial intelligence 173, 175, 179
    impact of 180
    intersection of 173
    powered telemedicine platforms 177
    role of 173, 176
Automated data extraction 178
Average axial length 95
Average deviation 72
Axial length 17, 24, 73t, 125t, 126t, 150
    groups 55, 59, 133
    scatter plots of 48f

B

Backup and data storage solutions 189
Bar diagram 42, 43f
Barrett true axial 46f
Barrett Universal II 46f
Best-corrected visual acuity 10, 19, 73, 137, 146, 208
    advantages of 19t
Bias mitigation 181
Binomial distribution 84
Bland-Altman plot 49, 50f
Blinding 195
    types of 195
Blood
    group types 15
    parameters 60
    pressure 34
    sugar levels 90
Bonferroni correction 9, 10t, 124
Bonferroni method 149, 152
Boxplots 46

C

Case-control study 203, 204, 204fc, 204t
Cataract surgery 67, 76f, 84, 99
Cell density 204
Central corneal thickness 204
Central foveal thickness 124
Central macular thickness 146

Central tendency 57, 60, 71
    measure of 53, 64, 66
Chi-square test 113, 132, 139
    applications of 114
    characteristics of 113
    validity of 114
Choroid 52
Choroidal changes 202t
Choroidal subfoveal thickness 135, 135t-137t
Choroidal vascularity index 10, 25
Chromatic adaptation 66
Clinical ophthalmology 193
Clinical tests 188
Cluster sampling 34, 35f, 38
Clustering, degree of 152
Cognitive load 6
Cohort study 203, 205fc, 205t
Color-coded images 50
Communication 183, 189
Comparative studies 70
Complex eye conditions 173
Composite series, mean of 56
Comprehensive statistical tools 167, 168
Confidence interval 109, 138, 139
Confounding bias 195, 195t
Conjunctivitis 63
    epidemic 63t
Consistency 57
Continuous learning 181
Continuous monitoring 175
Continuous probability distribution 85
    type of 85
Convenience sampling 36
Conventional fundus photography 95
Conventional phacoemulsification 73
Convolutional neural networks 177
Corneal curvature 125t, 126t
    radius 150
Corneal surgery, advanced visualization in 157
Corneal thickness 17, 88, 89, 118t
Corneal topography 50
Correlation
    analysis 90
    coefficient, measuring of 91
    types of 90
Coverage, depth of 5
COVID-19, blood parameters in 60
Cross-sectional study 200, 201
    design 201fc

Cumulative distribution functions 84
Curve, bell-shaped 87
Customer satisfaction surveys and market research 25

D

Data 13
    analysis 42, 161-164, 166-169, 173, 175, 176, 179, 213
    aspects of 161
    evolving field of 161
    phase 190
    plan 188
    ToolPak representation 163f
    tools in 161
    types of 64
    changes 61
    classification of 12, 12fc
    cleaning 162
    collection 5, 21, 22, 174, 176, 180
    challenges 178
    informants for 24
    methods 21-23, 183, 188
    phase 188
    sensor-based 189
    sources of 23b
    techniques 21
    confidentiality 189
    distribution of 65, 84
    kinds of 84
    management 166, 171
    measurement of 13
    methodical collection of 21
    organization 161
    preprocessing 174, 176
    processing 176
    representation 163f, 165
    requirement 61
    security 189
    serves 22
    set 53
    source 197
    type of 16
    validation 189
    verification 189
    visualization 5, 168, 169
Dataset, central value of 57
Deep capillary plexus 25, 135
Deep learning 177
Defocus incorporated multiple segments lens 145

Dependent variable 101, 127
Descemet's membrane endothelial
   keratoplasty 157
Descriptive statistics 5, 161, 164
   dialog box 164
Descriptive studies 198, 199
Designing
   fundamental aspects of 143
   study 174, 176
Diabetic retinopathy 71t, 73, 90,
   99, 177, 178
   early signs of 179
Diagnostic test
   accuracy of 153
   interpreting accuracy of 139
   performance metrics, steps in 138t
Diopters 145
Direct personal investigation 23
Disc center-fovea angle 95
Discrete probability distributions 84
Dispersion, measures of 69
Dissemination 191, 214
   plans 191
Distribution, types of 78, 84
Documentation 184, 191
Dry eye symptoms 94

E

Early treatment diabetic retinopathy
   study chart 186
Ecological studies 203
Educational research 164
Effective communication 183
Egger's test 210
Electronic health records 174
   use of 188
Electronic medical records 177, 196
Email 184
Empirical rule 87
Endothelial cell
   count 73t, 74
   density 73
Enumerators method 22, 23, 25
Epidemiological methods 196
Epidemiological studies 39, 83, 196
   classification of 196t
   effectiveness in 177
Epidemiology 195
Epiretinal membrane 73
Ethical aspects overview 6

Ethical considerations 5, 147, 181, 213
Ethical standards 4
Ethics committee 187, 213
Exclusion criteria 186
Experimental research 147
Exponential distribution 85
Extensive libraries 168
Extracapsular cataract extraction 19
Eye
   color 15, 85
   conditions, diagnosis of 83
   diseases 178
      causes of 177
      prevalence of 177
      type of 15
   examinations 31
   health, field of 104
   infections, incidence of 114
   pressure 97f

F

Farsightedness 88
Feasibility 187
Femtosecond laser-assisted cataract
   surgery 73, 73t, 74
Final data analysis 188
Fisher exact T-test 136
   applications of 137t
Flat corneal meridian 24
Flexibility 168
Flipping coin 82
Focus groups 26, 189
Forest plot 49, 51f
Foveal avascular zone 135, 137
Freedom, degree of 106, 119,
   125-127, 150
Friedman test 135, 136, 136t, 137t
F-statistic 121, 122, 127, 128
Fundamental techniques 104

G

Ganglion cell complex 55
   thickness measurements 55, 59
Gathering information
   methods of 22
   process of 22
Gaussian curve 87f
Gaussian distribution 86
Gaussian mixture models 173

General data protection
        regulation 187
Geometric mean 65
Glaucoma 83, 97f, 98, 99, 120, 177, 178
    prevalence of 34
    progression of 90
    severity of 15
    stage of 32
Glycated hemoglobin, negative linear
        relationship of 100f
Gold standard test 154
Graft
    detachment 157
    failure 157
Graphical representation 61, 162
Graphical user interface 164
Ground truth coverage rate 66
Groundbreaking research 21
Grouped data 54, 55, 59t, 58, 62

H

Handling complex
    data 167
    study designs 169
Handling epidemiologic data 169
Handling inter-eye correlation 170
Handling large datasets 168
Harmonic mean 66
Health research 164
Heat maps 49, 50
    use of 52
Heterogeneity assessment 210
Heterogeneous data 57
Hidden Markov models 173
High standard deviation 74
Histograms 43
Holistic clinician 1, 2t, 3, 8
Homogeneity 126
Horner's syndrome 43, 43f
Humphrey visual field 10
Hydrophobic biospheric monofocal
        intraocular lenses 26, 45
Hyperopia 88
Hypothesis 106, 107, 118, 119, 122, 127,
        209, 213
    testing 104, 106, 107, 151, 174, 175

I

Implementation project 183
Implementing simple random
        sampling 32

Inclusion criteria 186
Independent T test 117, 118, 145, 146
    importance of 118
Inferential statistics 5, 104, 105
Information bias 194, 194t
Informed consent 187
Initial data analysis 70
Innovations, impact of 215
Institutional review board 213
Intensive care unit 175
Interdisciplinary collaboration 1, 6
Interim analysis 188
International Labour Organization 28
International Monetary Fund 28
Interquartile range 46, 69
Interval data 16, 17b
Interviews 21, 23, 188
Intraocular lens 24
    power calculations, crucial
        role in 90
Intraocular pressure 10, 16, 17, 24, 64t,
        72, 73, 76f, 90, 137, 143
    distribution of 86
    readings 185, 186
Intraoperative optical coherence
        tomography, use of 157
Intravitreal antivascular endothelial
        growth factor injection,
        effect of 118t

J

Judgment sampling 35

K

Karl-Pearson correlation
        coefficient 91
Keratitis, infectious 82
Keratoconus, awareness of 201
Keratometry values, mapping of 51f
Kruskal-Wallis H test 80, 133, 133t,
        134, 134t
    applications of 134t
    importance of 134
Kurtosis
    high 78
    low 78
    medium 78
    test 77, 79
    types of 78, 78f

Index

L

Large-scale epidemiological studies 40
Laser in situ keratomileusis 115*t*, 117*t*
Leadership, guidance of 185
Lens thickness 89
Likelihood ratios, concept of 110
Likert scale 15*f*
Line graphs 47
Linear regression
    analysis 94, 95*f*, 95*t*
    line 92*f*
Literature
    review 185
    search and study selection 209
Logistic regression 96, 97*t*
    curve presenting 97*f*
    model estimates 97
LogMAR
    chart 18*f*, 19*t*
    visual acuity notation qualifies 19
Long eyes groups, mean absolute error for 46*f*
Longitudinal study 201, 202, 202*fc*, 202*t*
Low standard deviation 74

M

Machine learning 173, 175, 177
    models 67, 173
    tools, impact of 180
Macula hole 73
Macular degeneration 83, 99
Macular fovea choroidal perfusion 150
Macular retinal thickness 135, 136*t*, 137*t*
Mailing method 24
Main data, nature of 186
Mann-Whitney U test 80, 129, 130*t*
    applications of 130*t*
Manuscript
    final review of 191
    preparation 190, 214
Mathematical properties 57
McNemar's test, sample size for 155
Mean
    deviation 72, 87
    estimation of 153
    square 125, 126, 128, 150
Median
    classification of 57*f*
    computation of 58
    demerits of 61
    formula for 58
    merits of 61
    properties of 60
Medical degrees 1
Medical images, analysis of 177
Medical research 42
    integrating statistical methods in 102
Medical science, branch of 195
Medical tests 188
Meta-analysis 195*t*, 209*t*, 209
Methodological rigor 187
Meticulous design 210
Micro-bypass stent 47*f*
Microincision cataract surgery 9
Minimizing selection bias 38
Mode
    demerits of 64
    merits of 64
    properties of 64
Model building 173
Mood's median test 132, 132*t*, 134, 134*t*
Multimodal data, integration of 181
Multiple modes 64, 65
Multiple parameters 136*t*
    changes in 137*t*
Multiple regression 99
    analysis 100
    equation 101
Multivariate analysis 98, 98*t*
Myopia 23, 115
    severity 125, 150

N

Natural language processing 175, 177, 178
    enhances data collection 178
    extracts 177
Neovascular age-related macular degeneration 159
Nominal data 13, 15, 15*t*
Nonarteritic anterior ischemic optic neuropathy 9, 10
Non-numeric data 64, 65
Nonparametric tests 80, 128
Nonrandom sampling methods 30, 35
Nonrandomized clinical trial 206, 208*t*
Normal curve 87*f*
Normal distribution 85-87

Null hypothesis 107, 108, 117-119, 122, 126, 127, 155

O

Observation 188
Observational research 40
Observational studies 196, 198
  subtypes of 198
One-way analysis of variance
  sample size for 149
  technique 150t
  test 136, 136t, 137t
Ongoing collaborations, documentation of 192
Ophthalmic emergency 44, 44f
Ophthalmic statistics 173
Ophthalmological studies 176
Ophthalmology 39, 81, 164, 168, 170, 177, 179, 180
  advance understanding in 214
  applications in 99
  aspects of 83
  clinical research 37
  community 214
  data 129
    analysis in 166, 167, 169
    driven project in 183
  ever-evolving field of 21
  field of 21, 67
  fundamental measurement in 88
  realm of 113, 143
  research 39
    data analysis in 161
  sampling 37
Optic disc drusen 130
Optical aberrations 66
Optical coherence tomography 89, 101, 121, 208
  angiography 208
  scans 51
Ordinal data 13, 17b
Outer retinal layer 146

P

Pain
  post-surgery 15f
  degree of 15
Paired T-test 117, 119, 121t
  applications of 120t

Parametric tests 112, 113
Pars plana vitrectomy 73t
Pearson's correlation 93
Pediatric uveitis, visual outcomes of 20
Peripapillary choroidal thickness 10
Peripapillary microvasculature 102
Peripapillary vessel density, scatter plots of 100
Phacoemulsification 19, 47f, 205t
Phakic group 118
Pie chart 44, 45f
Pilot studies 148
Planning phase 185
Poisson distribution models 85
Polynomial indicates, degree of 95
Polynomial regression 95, 96b, 96f
  applications of 96
  second degree 95
Post COVID-19
  infection 135t, 136t, 137t
  morphometric changes in 135
Posterior capsule opacification 45
  severity of 26
Post-hoc tests 124, 128t, 129t
Post-laser assisted in situ keratomileusis surgery 23
Postsurgical intraocular pressure controls 47f
Post-test probability 110, 111
Power analysis 169
Pretest probability 110
Primary data 23, 27b
  collection 23
Probability 81-83
  density functions 84
  distributions 83
  formula for 82
  theory 173
Productive collaboration 192
Progressive visual deterioration 3
Pseudophakic eyes 19
Pseudophakic group 118
Public health
  interventions 101
  planning 83
Pulse rates 34
Pupil boundary, detection of 67
Pupil diameter 17
P-value 10, 19, 24, 55, 59, 60, 73, 79, 106, 111, 128, 130, 131, 133, 135, 137, 139, 145, 146

Q

Quadratic regression 95
Qualitative data 13
Quality control 70
Quality of life 99, 147
Quantitative data 16
Questionnaires 21, 24, 27, 188
Quota sampling 35

R

Random number generators 32
Random sampling 30, 31, 38
   methods 31
Random starting point 34
Randomization tools 32
Randomized clinical trials 155
Randomized control
   study 207t
   trials 206, 207
Rank data 16, 129
Real-world implementation 175
Refractive correction, quality of life
       impact of 145
Refractive error 88, 89
   measurements 16
Regression
   analysis 94, 102, 162, 175
      serves 102
      types of 94
   applications of 101
   equations 94
   technique 94
Reliability 167
Reproducibility 167, 168
Research
   degrees 1
   frameworks 193
   hypothesis 155
   institutions, publications of 28
   methodology 4, 180
   objective 183, 185
   project flow 212
   question 174, 208, 209
Resolution, minimum
       angle of 10, 73, 137
Retina 52
Retinal changes 202t
Retinal disease 3
Retinal nerve fiber layer 102, 120, 121, 130, 133
   thickness 89
      measurements 133
Retinal thickness 17, 96f
Retinitis pigmentosa 99, 130, 130t
Rhegmatogenous retinal detachment 73
Robust tests 78

S

Sample size 153-156, 158
   calculation 145t, 146t, 169, 186, 188
      basic concepts for 143
      techniques 159
   computation 145, 149
   determination 143
   preoperative descriptive
       statistics of 24
Sampling
   interval 32, 34
   methods 5, 30
   techniques 30, 39
   unique aspects of 37
Scatter plots 47, 48f, 100, 100f, 162
   use of 48
Scheff's test 124
Scientific Committee Rigor 187
Secondary data 27
   collection 23
Select data analysis 164
Selection bias 194, 194t
Sensitivity 57, 110, 134, 138, 139
Separate focus sessions
   importance of 4
   need for 5
Shapiro-Wilk test 79
Short eyes groups, mean absolute
       error for 46f
Significance, level of 144
Simple random sampling 31
Single vision lens 145
Skew test 79
Skewness 76
   negative 76, 88
   positive 76, 88
   right 88
Snellen chart 20t, 186
   clinical use 18f
Snellen visual acuity notation 18, 19

Snowball sampling 37
Social sciences
    statistical package for 164, 166, 179
    tool 165f
Spearman's correlation 93
    coefficient 92, 94
Specificity 110, 139, 154
Spectral domain anterior segment
        optical coherence tomography,
        role of 131
Spherical equivalent 24, 48f
    refraction 145
Sphericity 127
    assumption 151
Squares, sum of 125-127, 150
Standard deviation 24, 73-75, 87, 105
    values of 73t, 74
Standard therapy, existence of 158
Stata in statistical analysis in
        ophthalmology research,
        advantages of 170
Statistic 106, 175
    encompasses 12
    fundamental concept in 82, 87
Statistical analysis 4, 5, 86, 164, 181, 210
    artificial intelligence tools for 179
    essential in 70
    fundamental in 69
    system 166
        applicability of 166
        interface of 167f
    use in 75
Statistical distributions 89
Statistical inquiry 22
Statistical measure 77
Statistical methods 151, 173
    use of 1
Statistical package 164
Statistical significance 136
    tests, applications of 79t
Statistical technique 98
Statistical tests 139
Statistical tools 81
Statistician, specific role of 188
Steep corneal meridian 24
Stratified random sampling 32, 33f
Study
    assessing quality of 209
    design 4, 8, 155t, 183, 185, 188, 193,
        197, 197fc, 213
    protocols 39
    group 24
    objective 193
    participants, age of 54t
    population 194
    rationale 187
    type of 155, 185
Subfoveal choroidal thickness 146
Superficial capillary plexus 25, 135
Surgical procedure, success rate of 81
Survey 22, 27, 188
    data analysis 164
Swept-source optical coherence
        tomography 9, 10
Systematic random
        sampling 32, 33, 33f, 34

T

Tear film stability 94
Toric intraocular lens 50f
Trade associations, publications of 28
T-test 78, 86, 114, 117t, 131,
        131t, 147, 175
    application of 131
T-value 131
Two-way analysis of variance 124

U

Uncorrected visual acuity 128, 129
Ungrouped data 53, 54, 54t, 55, 58, 62
Uniform distribution 85, 147
United Nations Organization 28
User-friendly interface 168, 169, 171

V

Variable 79, 131, 137, 165f, 184, 186
Vascular endothelial growth factor 118
Versatility 168
Visual acuity 15, 18, 20, 56, 56t, 76f, 88
    baseline 56
    change in 20, 20t
    follow-up 56
    gradations in 20
    granular measurement of 19
    measurements 66, 74, 75t, 76, 88,
        185, 186
    representation of 20, 20t, 60
    scores 16
    values 93f

Visual analog scale 150
Visual field 130
    test 179
Visual function 99
Visual outcome 20, 84*t*
Visualization capabilities 167
Vital signs 34
Vulnerable populations 188

W

White-to-white distance 24
Wilcoxon signed rank test 129, 131, 132

Z

Zero skewness 76
Z-score 70
Z-values 144, 145